Love and Infertility

Love and Infertility

Survival Strategies for Balancing Infertility, Marriage, and Life

□   □   □

Kristen Magnacca

LifeLine
Press·

A Regnery Publishing Company, Washington, D.C.

Library of Congress Cataloging-in-Publication Data
Magnacca, Kristen.
Love and infertility: survival strategies for balancing infertility, marriage, and life / Kristen Magnacca.
  p. cm.
 Includes index.
 ISBN 0-89526-056-5
1. Infertility—Popular works. 2. Self-help techniques. I. Title.
 RC889.M333 2005
 616.6'92—dc22
                2004014247

Published in the United States by
LifeLine Press
A Regnery Publishing Company
One Massachusetts Avenue, NW
Washington, D.C. 20001

Distributed to the trade by
National Book Network
4720-A Boston Way
Lanham, Maryland 20706

Printed on acid-free paper

Manufactured in the United States of America

10 9 8 7 6 5 4 3 2 1

Books are available in quantity for promotional or premium use. Write to: Director of Special Sales, Regnery Publishing, Inc., One Massachusetts Avenue, NW, Suite 600, Washington, D.C. 20001, for information on discounts and terms or call (202) 216-0600.

The information contained in this book is not a substitute for medical counseling and care. All matters pertaining to your physical health should be supervised by a health care professional.

To my friend, husband, and soul mate, Mark, who makes my life complete; my wonderful son, Cole, who fills my life with joy, and to my daughter, Princess Grace Sarah Rose, my gifts from God.

In loving memory of Auntie Joanne Darcy Hewes, who taught me many of life's lessons and showed me the real meaning of "No Guts, No Glory;" and Sarah Anne Seaman Dubuque, whom I miss daily and thank for her eternal love and friendship.

contents

Part III: Rolling with the Changes

Love and Infertility

"We're pregnant and we weren't even trying!" My friend's voice boomed with excitement over the phone. "Yippee!" I responded, echoing her excitement.

I have heard that same statement from others, and I'm sure you have, too. That afternoon, my thoughts ran to similar conversations I'd had with other friends, and I arrived at this conclusion: There are three groups of couples that enter into parenthood.

Group One: The "One Enchanted Evening" Pregnancy Group

The night was just perfect: Probably a romantic dinner for two, music on the stereo, some nice wine (perhaps a bit too much wine), and then a sexy romp under the covers to round out the night. A few weeks later, you're feeling tired and, almost as an afterthought, you take a home pregnancy test and find that you're with child. Just one enchanted evening, and bingo! You're pregnant!

Group Two: Your Basic,
Average Pregnancy Group

First there's one enchanted evening, then maybe an attempt to recreate the one-enchanted-evening experience, and still no success. You and your partner start to pay attention to the "signs" that indicate you're at your peak fertility and have intercourse at the appropriate times. Two or three months go by, and still no success. Then you give it the good ole' college try for three more months, and voilà—success! The average couple takes six months to conceive a child. Sometimes it's great to be average!

Group Three: The "Oh, My Goodness,
I Think We Have a Problem" Group

You've done the "one enchanted evening" thing, you've progressed through the average category, trying really, really hard, and still no success. Then you realize that it's the *anniversary* of your enchanted evening. It's been a whole year and no success. Anxiety and fear creep in. You go to see your obstetrician/gynecologist, who does the right thing and refers you to a reproductive endocrinologist. The expert informs you that, yes, unfortunately, you are one of the one in six couples who have unprotected sex for a year and have not achieved pregnancy: You're infertile. Ouch.

My husband, Mark, and I were firmly entrenched in Group Three before we conceived our son, Cole. We experienced the one enchanted evening and the desire to create that experience again and again to conceive naturally. Then we progressed through the six-month average club. Ultimately, we landed soundly in Group Three, where we remained for another three years. After Cole's birth, even while drawing on our professional lives and our personal experiences from our first attempts, we tried for our second child and again found ourselves in Group Three. But we never gave up hope that the magic of just one enchanted evening might work for us. It was a journey filled with bumps and bruises, but we made it to the finish line and welcomed our daughter, Grace, into our family.

Infertility is difficult, scary, overwhelming, and, at times, heartbreaking. It took Mark and me eight years of trying very, very hard before we finally created our family. As a couple, we experienced what every relationship goes through, but our ups and downs were made more intense by our desperate desire to have a family and the wrenching physical, emotional, and spiritual issues we faced as we struggled with our inability to conceive.

Mark and I make our living by helping people do and be their best. We founded and run a successful corporate consulting company, Insight Development Group, Inc. We specialize in creating seminar experiences designed to help people expand what they believe is possible.

As we struggled against infertility, it dawned on us: Why not apply our corporate training concepts to the issues we were facing in our marriage? So little by little, we started putting into practice the strategies, exercises, tips, and tricks we use in our seminars. We used our negotiating skills to assure that each of our needs were met. We played simple games and did easy exercises to help us communicate better. We also made tough choices as we learned to compromise lovingly and selflessly.

It worked.

So my purpose in writing this book is to share with you these proven strategies to help you effectively communicate with your spouse or partner, maintain a sense of control over your lives, and help you deal with the changes associated with the process of becoming parents.

Love and Infertility is designed like a full buffet. One strategy might resonate with you today, whereas another might not be as appealing. For me, when I'm at a buffet, I hardly ever take olives for my salad, but on some days I plop one on the top and that olive just hits the spot. Today you might not feel like trying one particular strategy, but maybe next week it will be your olive and really hit the spot. I encourage you to use the book as a buffet or menu, picking a strategy that fits the needs of your current situation.

It can be tricky to keep a sense of balance while you deal with infertility, nourish your marriage, and live out your daily life. The strategies in this book are designed to help you keep that sense of balance and perspective as you strive to create your family.

I

Creating Your Destiny

The Dreams List

When Mark and I were trying to have a baby, the "trying to have a baby" part became my sole focus. Okay, I was obsessed, and with my obsession came a loss of priority, spinning me totally out of balance—mind, body, and soul.

I wasn't thinking about myself as a whole person; I was just "Kristen Magnacca, trying to have a baby." My life revolved around *trying* to create our baby, and the energy of *trying* to create a baby is what I was presented with each and every day. I was, in a sense, creating a reality of *trying*. My actions, thoughts, and desires were consumed with *trying*, and I was stuck *trying*, not *creating*. I was simply sending the wrong intention out into the universe and getting back the same unhealthy energy I was sending out.

I believe that controlling how you send your intention out into the universe is the most important act that you can do in your life.

How do you send your intentions out and receive your desired outcome? It is as easy as answering this question: *If I had unlimited time, talent, money, and support from my family, what would I do with my life?*

If this is your introduction to goal-setting, I understand if you're feeling a little skeptical. So was I when Mark first introduced me to this exercise years ago.

It all started in a Florida airport. Mark and I had taken a long weekend to celebrate my birthday in combination with a work engagement. I was at the airport, getting ready to fly home. Mark was going to wrap up his business, then fly home a few days later.

The plane began to board and I turned to collect my carry-on pieces. As I fumbled with my bags and tickets, Mark handed me a card and a small box. "Open the card on the plane, but open the box now," he said. In the box was a sterling silver bracelet, which I quickly put on my wrist. I had a flash of confusion about why he had waited to give me such a special gift at such a hectic moment.

As we said our goodbyes, tears began to fall. "Call me when you land and I'll see you in a few days," Mark said. His voice was soft and strong.

We had only been a "couple" for six months, and we were coming to the realization that each of us had found our soul mate.

After taking my window seat on the plane, I clipped my seatbelt together and stored my bag under the seat in front of me like a dutiful traveler. I was settled in for the three-hour flight up the East Coast to Massachusetts. When I opened the card, a ragged piece of notebook paper with Mark's handwriting on it fell out onto my lap. The first line read: *"If I had unlimited time, talent, money, and support from my family, here is a list of all the things I would do with my life."* I put the birthday card down and opened the well-worn paper. The date in the upper-right-hand corner showed this had been written almost one year before. What was this all about?

My confusion grew as I began reading a laundry list of attributes: *I would spend my life with my partner, who would:*

- ✿ possess a keen mind and good attitude
- ✿ have a good sense of humor
- ✿ be 100 percent loyal
- ✿ have a cheerful, sunny disposition
- ✿ love to converse about everything
- ✿ know how to enjoy silence...

After reading each number, my inner voice responded, "That's me!" and then the enormity of this small, well-worn piece of paper hit me. By the time I got to number sixteen, I was in a full-blown crying spell. I was holding Mark's vision or "Dreams List" for his ideal soul mate and, fortunately for me, I was an exact match. My eyes were beginning to swell and I was audibly gasping for breath. The little non–English-speaking grandmother sitting next to me became visibly uncomfortable; touching my arm, she offered me a cookie. Wiping my nose, I shook my head "no" in response.

I was overcome with the shock of how accurately I was described (I'm not as conceited as this might sound) by Mark before we had even met. He had put down his ideal image of the woman who would be his spouse and sent it out into the universe and, in doing so, he found me and I found him!

That was my introduction to the powerful exercise of writing down intentions. It was, in effect, a mission statement for his marriage partner, and he was able to manifest *us*.

When our relationship progressed from the dating stage to engagement, we began designating January 1 of each year as the day we'd come together in sweatpants and bed-head and create our vision for the next year by answering that same simple question: "*If*

I had unlimited time, talent, money, and support from my family, what would I would do with my life?"

Years later, we were engulfed in the confusion and frustration of trying to have a baby, and we realized we had forgotten how this powerful strategy had helped us make so many of our collective dreams realities. The simple act of writing our intentions down on paper always seemed to open up a new realm of possibilities.

After Mark and I lost our first pregnancy (it was an ectopic pregnancy), I fell rapidly to a place of despair and darkness. A place that I had no idea existed—and I didn't have the skills needed to climb out!

I thought I had two choices: The first was to stay in our darkened bedroom and shrivel up and be mad at everyone in the world, including God. The second was to do something to honor our lost baby.

We decided to do what we had always done, something that had worked so well in our past, until we stopped doing it for some unknown reason. With paper and pen in hand, we created a new "Dreams List." This started a chain reaction that helped us go from the depths of despair to literally making our dreams a reality again.

That New Year's Day, after completing our joint "Dreams List," we narrowed the list down to the top three most important goals for the next year for each of us. My three goals were:

- ❀ Be a mom
- ❀ Publish *Girlfriend to Girlfriend: A Fertility Companion*
- ❀ Be on the *Today Show* to bring national awareness to the issue of infertility

My goals sent Mark into a semi-panic. I was a broken, fertility-challenged woman who had just lost a baby, had never written nor published a book, and really had no idea how to get on to the number-one morning news show! But those were attainable goals to me. With my faith in the universe and God, I set out on my yearly tasks.

I chose a purple 3x5 card, wrote down my new goals in my best possible penmanship, and tucked the card into my day-runner. This simple act helped remind me of my goals and gave me a quiet confidence.

The following year was hectic but focused. As the months clicked away, we were working on becoming parents biologically and through adoption. At the same time, I had completed my manuscript and was in the process of having the book published.

Mark was cautiously optimistic and very gentle with me regarding my *Today Show* aspirations. He walked a fine line between being supportive and realistic. "Kristen, you know that even with the most well-known public relations firms, it takes a lot of hard work and effort to get national coverage on any story," Mark said in a sweet, yet firm, tone. Then, one day in October, I was working at my desk and received a call from my friend and mentor Dr. Ali Domar.

During our crisis period, I had attended her well-known and innovative mind/body infertility program located in the Boston area. When Mark realized that I was slipping away into the great darkness of depression, he had tried to get help for our marriage and me. A friend told him about Dr. Domar, and he frantically called to get me into the program.

Meeting Dr. Domar was a turning point for me. I frequently refer to her as my "angel of light" because she helped me bring my life back into balance.

Dr. Domar was calling that day to ask me for a favor. She wasn't able to make a promotional date for her new book that was coming out in November, and she wanted to know if I'd be willing to go on the *Today Show* to tell my story and share my experience with her program.

I was in total shock but immediately answered, "Yes, I would!"

The enormity of the phone call did not hit until I was in the elevator going down to take my place on the couch to be interviewed. Upon entering NBC's Studio 1A, I felt as though I had to hold myself together and speak for all the couples who were currently in the process of trying to have a baby. I thought to myself, "How did I get here?" and realized this was the manifestation of that neatly written statement on my purple 3x5 card.

This experience was an enormous life lesson for me. I had the determination and faith that this goal would happen, and I had been visualizing this outcome. The lesson I learned was that the manifestation of this goal did not happen in the manner that I had expected—that the roads by which we reach our goals are not always the ones we have chosen. This made me think about our baby situation as well. I realized that I held on so tightly to my preconceived notion of how our dream of a family would be manifested that I was constraining any other possibilities. In other words, I was blindly determined to be in Group One: the "one enchanted evening" group!

This life experience opened me up to the idea that by releasing an intention into the universe, you are tapping into a level of awareness at which all things are possible if you are willing to give up your idea of how you will get to your outcome.

Putting It into Practice

There are two parts to this strategy. It's important that you do both of them to maximize your chances of getting the universe to hear your intentions.

Take out a loose sheet of paper (or you may want to purchase a strategy notebook to keep your answers to the strategies organized).

On that sheet of paper, write down the following statement:

If I had unlimited time, talent, money, and support from my family, here is a list of all the things I would do with my life for the next twelve months.

For the next five minutes, simply let your thoughts "pop" from your mind onto your paper. Don't concern yourself about how outrageous your desires might be, just let them pour out. Be sure to state your responses in the present tense and in a positive manner.

Here are a few examples to get you started:

- Be a mom
- Give birth to a healthy baby
- Create a healthy environment for myself and my baby
- Take dance classes
- Plant an herb garden
- Redecorate our living room in earth tones

Congratulations! You have just officially joined the elite five percent of the population who have written down their goals for the future.

Now follow up that exercise with the second part of the strategy.

Review your list and choose the top three goals that you want to complete in the next twelve months.

I recommend that you then take a 3x5 notecard (I use the eye-catching colored index cards) and date the card in the right-hand corner. Then number one to three on the left. On the first line, write down the goal that you believe is your first priority, and follow that with your second priority and then your third priority.

I encourage you to put your card in a place that you'll notice regularly. Mark keeps his in his wallet; I keep mine in my day-runner. You don't need to take them out and read them every single day, but just having them in a place that you notice regularly makes things happen.

This exercise can and will have a profound impact on your life. By focusing clearly on your future dreams and desires, you can present the universe with the correct direction to make all things possible.

Motivational speaker Napoleon Hill said that your mind cannot tell the difference between something vividly imagined and a real experience. That's why our dreams are so powerful. That concept resonated well with me, and I think it'll resonate with you, too.

According to Hill, *"Anything your mind can conceive and believe, you can achieve."*

The Fertility Game Plan

I'm going to let you in on a little secret—a somewhat embarrassing secret. When Mark's and my premarital relationship progressed to a more serious level of intimacy, contraception became an almost competitive issue. We were both vying for control; neither of us would relinquish our own preferred method of protection. I'm not sure if this is common with all type-A individuals or just with us, but I was taking birth control pills daily and Mark wore a condom every time we made love. In retrospect, our extreme measures were pretty comical, in a twisted way, given the heartbreaking challenge that procreation would soon become.

It wasn't until we were married and happily installed in our new Boston-area home that we loosened our control. After all, the plan was to start creating a family as soon as the dust settled from the move. Or at least that's what I thought.

One crisp New England winter day, shortly after the dueling contraceptives had been cast aside, a casual stroll through the woods behind our house gave way to a startling discovery. Out of the blue, Mark blurted out that he was having second thoughts and wasn't sure he was ready to have a baby. "Maybe I'm not ready for this next step yet," he said.

I was floored! We had discussed having children, and the plan was for me to sell my business, sell my house, move in with him, and instantly become pregnant! Now that I had fulfilled my part of the bargain, my new husband appeared to be backpedaling on his.

"What are you talking about, Mark?" I raised my voice, startling some fluffy white snow from its peaceful perch on a tree branch above us.

"Well," he said, brushing the snow off his coat, "I was just thinking that maybe we should wait a year or so."

Truly, I could have hurt him at that moment! But I tried to practice reflective listening, which involves mirroring back what someone has said in order to communicate your understanding. (More to come about reflective listening as a communication tool in Strategy Sixteen.)

"So, let me get this straight," I said. "I think you're saying *you want to wait a year to have a baby!!!*"

My attempt at reflective listening was really more like screaming back at Mark what he just said to me. The enchantment of the forest was gone and so was my calm, cool state.

"I'm going home!" I trudged off, crunching the snow angrily beneath my feet.

This conversation was revisited again and again. I really did understand Mark's apprehension about taking this giant step to fatherhood. After all, I had my doubts about my own parenting abilities. But even when my fears bubbled to the surface, I never thought of discarding the plan. I was older than Mark and, for me, the timing was right.

A few days later, Mark invited me for another walk in the forest, and as soon as the words left his lips, I knew he wanted to clear the air about the baby conversation. As I bundled up against the frosty winter weather, I prepared myself for a more cool-headed, open-minded approach to this impending discussion.

"Mark, I've been thinking. If you feel that this isn't the 'right' time for us to have a baby, then I need to accept that. I'm so disappointed, though, and in some way feel as if I was bamboozled. I held up my part of the agreement and now you're renegotiating your side and changing the agreement altogether.

"I've been giving this new information a great deal of thought and have to let you know that I'm at a crossroads in my life now because of your change of mind. I had envisioned a child to love and devote myself to, but lately I've been thinking that I would like to start another company, and, if this is the route that I go, I won't be in a position to think about having a baby for the next five years. It's all or nothing for me, and you know that starting up any business takes one hundred percent of one's attention. So, you're right—our timing is off, and we should wait to start our family."

My monologue, of course, was pure garbage. I was using reverse psychology. Now, I don't know if my plan of attack worked or if Mark had reversed his opinion on his own before my devious little speech, but by the end of this second walk, both sides were in agreement: Now was the time to start a family.

This type of exchange—a dialogue fueled by our differing expectations—recurred throughout our months spent trying to conceive, especially when the stress of a high-pressure, high-tech fertility treatment was thrown into the already volatile emotional mix.

I had expected Mark to view the situation through Kristen-colored glasses, but he could only view it through his own. For example, when we were still hovering in the "average" pregnancy group, I had great concerns about the months ticking away, yet Mark seemed oblivious to any urgency. My interruption of his easygoing approach to our baby-making caused stress for both of us. While I wanted us to go to the doctor right away and start the testing process, he wanted to wait. I viewed every passing babyless day as wasted time, yet he thought we were just getting started. Six months to me was a lifetime of trying; six months to Mark was just a few times at bat. (He frequently used the baseball metaphor when referring to our baby-making. I did my best not to take offense.)

After a few of these back-and-forth discussions, it occurred to me that we work much better as a team when we have clear direction and understanding of each other's perception, position, and needs. Plans are most effective when they're in writing, hence the Fertility Game Plan.

Strategy Two—creating a Fertility Game Plan—is very important for couples trying to conceive. Mark and I developed ours for two reasons:

- ✿ To align our expectations, allowing us to work as a team from the same page and in the same direction

- ✿ To give us something concrete on which to focus while we were dealing with the abstract concept of creation

Mark and I kept at creating our family for years and had moments of heartbreak and times of triumph. During one particularly difficult period, while working toward our first child, a miscarriage due to an ectopic pregnancy pushed us to our breaking point. We knew that our goal of creating a family was still strong, but, in order to succeed, the game plan needed to be changed dramatically. To accommodate our newfound needs and desires, we totally revamped our game plan. The high-tech alternatives were our best route to conception, but we were also embracing the idea of adoption, and our plan had to reflect this.

Here is the Fertility Game Plan we used while trying for our first baby.

Mission: To become parents within twelve months from our first intrauterine insemination.

Agreement: Mark and Kristen are committed to attending all appointments together to provide an additional set of ears for obtaining information.

We also commit to the following actions:

- After receiving the nightly medication instructions from the clinic, Kristen will prepare her nightly hormone injections
- Mark will administer the nightly injections to Kristen at 6:30 P.M
- We will continue on a course of three intrauterine inseminations
- We will take a monthly break between each cycle
- We will take the summer months off
- We will progress to one cycle of in vitro fertilization (IVF) if necessary
- We will explore the option of adoption immediately, call three agencies, and attend their informational meetings
- Each of us will attend the orientation/informational adoption meetings
- We will schedule an appointment with a private adoption attorney

* We will plan a weekly date night where we do not discuss our fertility challenges

Mutual consent is necessary to modify this agreement.

Our son, Cole, was born on September 21, 1998. Because of our bumpy fertility journey, almost immediately after his birth we decided to try for another baby. We had learned from our earlier experience conceiving Cole what worked for us as a couple and what we needed to discuss and commit to on paper. For our daughter, Grace, who came into the world five long years after her brother, our mission and our agreement remained the same, but we needed to adapt our Fertility Game Plan slightly to fit our circumstances at the time. Our thorough planning for conceiving Gracie helped us maintain mutual understanding and respect throughout our attempts at conception. We relied on what we know now that we wished we had known then! Here's our activity commitment list from our second-time-around Fertility Game Plan.

* We will schedule an appointment with a reproductive endocrinologist
* If at all possible, we both will attend doctor's appointments together—four ears are better than two!
* Kristen will continue to receive craniosacral therapy and acupuncture treatments
* Kristen will take folic acid supplements
* Mark will wear boxer shorts, not briefs
* Kristen will have a repeat hysterosalpingogram
* Mark will visit the urologist and have a repeat semen analysis
* We agree to three rounds of in vitro fertilization

❀ If all of the above does not result in another miracle baby, we will be thankful to God for our family of three

This Fertility Game Plan was short and to the point, and still we had to revisit some issues. Mark felt I was too far on the alternative therapy side of working toward balance. He couldn't understand my reluctance to go full force with the Western medical approach. This caused some marital discussion, and renegotiations occurred regularly.

Putting It into Practice

The Fertility Game Plan exercise will provide you with a tool for discussion and allow for issues to be aired and overcome quickly. Here's how to get started on your own Fertility Game Plan. The exercises below are just a beginning point for discussion and creating your plan. I'm sure once you get started, your conversation will evolve and so will your plan.

You'll need two clean sheets of paper and your partner/spouse. Answer the following questions individually and then discuss your answers together:

❀ I envision our pregnancy to be

_____.

❀ I envision our life with a child to be

_____.

❀ I see myself as this kind of mom or dad

_____.

List three things that you feel you need during this time of creating a family.

1.

2.

3.

If we try for _____ months with no success, are you willing to seek medical intervention? What does this mean to you, and why?

If we are referred to a reproductive endocrinologist, are you willing to use assisted reproductive technologies to create a family?

If you are currently on the high-tech fertility treatment track, here are some important additional questions for you to discuss and to consider addressing in your game plan.

- Would you use donor sperm?

- Would you use donor eggs?

- How many eggs would you implant?

- Would you selectively reduce?

- What are your thoughts about assisted hatching?

- Would you consider a surrogate mom?

- What are three things you expect from each other if ever you find yourselves in a critical situation such as an ectopic pregnancy or a miscarriage?

- What would be your stopping point?

- What strategies for compromise would you implement if this stopping point were not agreed upon?

- Would you consider adoption?

Our Fertility Game Plan brought us both peace of mind and offered us strength as a couple. Just as with Strategy One: The Dreams List, once you get clear as a couple on how you'd like the baby-making experience to be, the universe will process your intention and help you move forward.

The Power of Visualization

One bright morning I stumbled into our master bathroom and, with my right eye open just a slit, started to line my toothbrush with toothpaste. All of a sudden, out of the fuzzy corner of my eye, I noticed a yellow sticky-note stuck to the mirror.

Although I am regarded in some circles as the Sticky-Note Queen, this time it wasn't me doing the sticking.

I opened both eyes as wide as they could possibly open at 6:00 AM and read a purple number 11 staring back at me from the little yellow square. I was confused. Why had Mark stuck the note there, and what was the significance of the 11?

That evening, while I was preparing dinner, Mark came in and began munching on the carrots I had out for the salad.

"Where did you have to be at eleven o'clock today?" I asked him.

"Hmmm?" Mark replied between crunches of carrot.

"At eleven—did you have to be somewhere at eleven?"

"No." He gave me a confused look and kept on munching.

"You left a sticky-note on the mirror with 'eleven' on it."

Mark started laughing around the carrot stick. "No, not *eleven o'clock*; it's not an eleven, it's a positive pregnancy test!"

Now I had the confused look on my face. Mark explained: "I watched Jim Carrey's biography last night and it reminded me again about the importance of visualization. I taped it for you—it's exactly what we talk about in our seminars. Nicolas Cage was on it, and Jim Carrey's sister. They told how Jim Carrey wrote himself a check for ten million dollars for 'acting services rendered,' post-dated it, and put it in his wallet. He carried it around with him for three years. Here's the amazing part: By the date on the check, he was worth the ten million. How incredible is that?"

"That gives me goose bumps," I replied.

"It was a motivating story, so when it was over, I drew two purple lines on the sticky-note and put it on the mirror so that every morning when I visualize our coming pregnancy, I can see the positive test result we're longing for," he said.

"You are so sexy to me right now," I said with a wink.

"That's why I married you, baby, because this stuff turns you on!" By this time we both were laughing.

Visualization is a mental rehearsal or vision of future events, and it's a powerful strategy to incorporate into your life. Peak performers in business use it, as do actors and Olympic athletes. And it's easy and cheap, too! Mark and I both utilized this technique and it helped both of us tremendously. There are, in fact, two versions of this visualization strategy. Mark's technique, creative visualization, was to actually visualize the positive result he was hoping to get. Jim Carrey's technique, while similar, is what we call "Acting As If." Let's take a closer look at these two techniques.

Creative Visualization

When I was undergoing fertility treatments, each morning I would visualize my blood being drawn pain-free. In my mind's eye, I would see myself walking into the clinic, sitting in the chair, and pulling up my sleeve. In my head, I saw the nurse wrap the cuff around my arm, and swab my forearm with alcohol to sterilize it, then watched the needle slip into my arm easily and without pain. Then, when the nurse was finished taking my blood sample, I saw myself bending my arm to stop the bleeding and the nurse applying the bandage. Bim, bam, boom—finished in a flash, without pain.

The actual scene so closely resembled how I visualized it that my nerves were calm and my whole body relaxed. Through mental rehearsal, I had, in a sense, already performed the task and knew how it turned out.

Visualization gives you a sense of control about things that are somewhat out of your control, and increases your comfort level regarding new things.

Another example, as it applies to creating our children, is a trick I would use when Mark and I were making love and trying to conceive. I would visualize Mark's sperm traveling trouble-free through my cervix, up into my fallopian tubes, and swimming their way to my uterus, where they would meet up with my freshly ovulated, grade-A egg and fertilize it within seconds.

"Acting As If"

When struggling young actor Jim Carrey wrote himself a check for ten million dollars, he was *acting as if* he were already an actor who was paid ten million dollars per picture. Mark and I adopted the Acting As If strategy, too, as it pertained to our creating a child.

We pretended and acted as if we were pregnant, to provide the best possible pre- and postconception environment for our unborn child. Acting As If is one aspect of creating your baby that you can control.

Putting It into Practice

Creative Visualization

The act of pre-playing events in your mind, and seeing yourself achieving the positive result you want, is a highly effective technique. When you recognize that an upcoming event is causing you to feel anxious, overwhelmed, or frightened, you can relieve these feelings by taking the following steps:

- ✿ Sit quietly for a few minutes and think about what event you'd like to mentally rehearse or practice.
- ✿ Begin to write your own mental screenplay in your mind's eye for the event you are about to rehearse. For example, maybe you have chosen your initial meeting with a reproductive endocrinologist. Your fear about this next step is almost debilitating. You might want to start out by imagining yourself leaving your house, getting into your car, arriving safely, checking in at the receptionist window, and so on. You are creating a situation in which you can trigger familiar, comfortable feelings where there are typically uncomfortable ones.
- ✿ Replay your screenplay over and over again, editing out as you go the portions that you feel you no longer need.

❧ Ask yourself questions as you move through the screenplay to help relieve negative emotions and create a beneficial "mental experience." For example, zero in on the one act or moment that is causing you the most discomfort.

❧ Ask yourself: What part of this upcoming event is most troubling to me? How can I manage this exchange in a way that will get the goal met and relieve my stress? The purpose of this mental rehearsal is to provide you comfort in place of fear of the unknown.

"Acting As If"

Here's how you can start "Acting As If":

For women

❧ Schedule an appointment with your obstetrician that includes a breast exam and a Pap smear.

❧ At your OB/GYN appointment tell your doctor and/or midwife that you're starting to create your family. Get their input regarding prenatal vitamins and folic acid.

For men

❧ Schedule an appointment for a complete physical.

❧ To increase sperm mobility and morphology and "turn down the heat in the kitchen," so to speak, switch from tighter briefs to loose boxers. It really makes a difference.

❧ Avoid hot tubs for the same reason.

For women and men

❧ Make it a point to eat a well-balanced diet that includes plenty of fresh vegetables and fruits, and be sure to get your daily allowance of calcium. These are easy changes to make and they're greatly beneficial to the little one in the making.

✿ Avoid extremes of exercise. Studies tell us that extreme exercise can decrease the progesterone levels in women; it's all about balance. Walk instead of run or cut down the number of miles that you walk or run; take yoga instead of aerobics. When you are in a treatment cycle it is best to have a discussion with your reproductive endocrinologist regarding your exercise regimen. It's about moderation and creating an environment that is conducive for conception.

✿ Avoid or cut down on alcoholic beverages. Try fresh juices with sparkling water or iced herbal teas with a little zing of lemon or lime. You can mix white or rosé wine with sparkling water for a wine cooler.

✿ If you haven't quit smoking yet, now's the time. Your family doctor or OB/GYN can give you lots of encouragement and advice on how to quit. If you can't quit, at least try to reduce the number of cigarettes you smoke daily.

✿ Avoid or cut down on caffeine. Gradually switch to decaf coffee (a quick switch may bring on that "caffeine withdrawal" headache), or try out some of the delicious new flavors of herbal teas. Decaffeinated sodas are also ubiquitous these days.

It was easy for me to get obsessive about not having alcohol, drinking caffeine-free beverages, and eating appropriately until I realized that, as in all parts of life, it's important to keep a balance. Mark and I kept a balance by periodically taking a break from "Acting As If." Taking a little time off from this strategy made it easier to keep up our commitment level.

four

Schedule Lamenting Time

We had been trying to get pregnant for months, with no success, and the process was wearing on my personality and work ethic.

I was so easily distracted during the day. Hour after hour, I was obsessing—thinking about the time of month, my fertility signals, and the likelihood of creating a baby during each month's attempt. I was driving myself nuts with all these thoughts. I think of each thought in my head as a person on my mental bus. The strongest thought at any given time sits behind the steering wheel and drives the bus, sometimes to a point of no return. It went something like this:

"Gee, I wonder if I took my folic acid today. I can't remember. Well, I'd better go and take one—or another one— just in case."

Working out of my home office was a curse and a blessing during these mental bus rides: Up the stairs to the kitchen to get the folic acid, back downstairs to the office.

"Okay, folic acid taken. What's today's date? Oh, that would be the tenth day of my cycle; the ovulation kit still only gave us one line. I wonder if there's a problem, I should retake the test."

And on and on and on it went.

Fear was the basis of all my internal conversations. I allowed my fear of not being able to get pregnant to permeate my thoughts and my day. This is where Strategy Four saved my days. It can save yours, too.

I began to "schedule" lamenting time. During the day, if a thought popped into my head, before I allowed that thought to climb behind the wheel, take control of the bus, and drive me to distraction, I would quickly jot it down on a colored sticky-note, and then stick it to my computer. (This was an appropriate place for me because I was isolated in my own home office, but this might not be the best for you, depending upon your individual situation.)

I would repeat this during the day, stopping, jotting the thought down, and then moving forward on my work to-do list. This strategy became powerful for a few reasons. First, I felt as though *I* was taking control of the emotional surge—and my mental bus—through the act of jotting the thought down on the piece of paper. Second, I felt as though I was giving it some acknowledgment for that brief moment. Having done that, I was then quickly able to regroup and maintain control of my workday. But this was only the first part of the strategy.

At the end of my workday, when all my other responsibilities were taken care of, I would allow myself fifteen minutes to focus on all the thoughts I had written down on those sticky-notes that day. I would review the notes and allow all the emotions contained on that colored paper to pour out. On some occasions I would cry in frustration at not being able to conceive. Other times I would laugh out loud at how outrageous the notes were and be thankful no one else was privy to my crazy thoughts! Either through laughter or through tears, I'd be releasing my emotions and making room in my system for new energy and new thoughts.

Mark, on the other hand, seldom resorted to this technique. He was able to compartmentalize the different aspects of his life: When he was at work, he worked, and when he was at play, he played. His ability to do this bothered me so much that it was frequently one of the thoughts I jotted down on a sticky-note and saved for the appropriate lamenting time.

Putting It into Practice

This technique is perfect for controlling fear and mental chatter, and will give you a chance to balance your emotions throughout the day. The goal of this strategy is to give yourself permission to feel what you need to feel, but at an appropriate time. Allowing yourself to feel helps your body purge itself of negative and toxic emotions.

Part One: The List

* You'll need a piece of paper, or a notepad, or a stack of little pieces of paper. (As you already know, I recommend those little colored sticky-notes.)

* Keep this paper and a pen or pencil nearby throughout the day.

* Whenever a stray thought pops into your head, quickly write it down on your notepad or on a separate sheet of paper.

✿ Repeat this step during the day, stopping, jotting the thought down, and then moving forward with whatever task you have at hand.

Part Two: Schedule Lamenting Time

✿ At the end of each day, after compiling your list of stray, distracting thoughts, set aside fifteen minutes when you know you won't be disturbed.

✿ Now review your list, allowing yourself to feel the emotions that each thought brings up for you. Focus on that thought alone, permit yourself to experience the excitement, or grief, or sadness, or disappointment—whatever the emotion. Then move on to the next "thought" on your list or in your pile of notes.

✿ Move through your list until you've addressed each "thought."

✿ Feel the release of tension and the toxic "obsessing." You should feel lighter, less distracted, and better able to focus on what tomorrow will bring.

For me, working this exercise was like giving myself the gift of freedom and the permission to feel without guilt.

I encourage you to give yourself the gift of fifteen minutes during the day to think, purge, and release all the harmful energy that is stored with negative emotions. And just think what a wonderfully positive environment you are creating for your baby!

five

Take a Mental Vacation

Okay, it's been one of those days when you haven't had an opportunity to use the bathroom since before you left the house this morning. Your shoulders are pulled up so high around your ears that you can't hear clearly, and your jaw is clamped so tightly that you have to remind yourself to relax it just to answer the phone.

Your body has been invaded by stress. You need to find serenity— and fast.

Strategy Five: Take a Mental Vacation, is a great way to shake off the pressures of your day and relieve your stressed body. You can take a mental vacation—a controlled, out-of-body experience achieved through visualizing a place of comfort or relaxation—any time, no matter where you are.

I began taking mental vacations when I was running my own company, but I used them more extensively when I was in fertility treatments. On the day of our second intrauterine insemination (IUI), it became apparent that it was not going to be an easy procedure for me.

The nurse was apparently unfamiliar with the procedure and was having a terrible time pushing the catheter filled with Mark's sperm through my cervix. Finally, she called a second nurse in for backup. Meanwhile, my fight-or-flight response was kicking in, and I was definitely leaning toward flight. I just wanted to run away from the situation altogether.

But obviously I couldn't, because this procedure was the most important part of the IUI, and despite my discomfort, I knew I had to go through with it. So I took a mental vacation. I allowed myself to travel to a beach that I had visited when I was in St. Croix. Closing my eyes and thoughts to the unpleasant goings-on around me, I drifted to a place where sun shined on the crystal-clear ocean, where the mountains met the sea. I visualized myself seated in a chair under two palm trees that had grown toward each other, criss-crossing at the top. The breeze blowing by cooled the hot sun on my skin, and the ice in my drink clinked against the side of the glass while I took a sip. Sitting on the beach in my mind's eye, I was able to soothe the fight-or-flight response rushing through my body. For those short minutes, I was accomplishing two things: I created a sense of peace in my body, and I permitted myself to do exactly what I wanted to do—"run away" from it all yet still be able to complete the task at hand. It was a perfect escape.

When I was delivering my daughter, Grace, I relied on my mental vacation to get me through the stages of labor, and I was able to manage the pain drug-free using this strategy of visualizing St. Croix. I also called on another short mental movie I had learned from my friend Dr. Ali Domar. The shorter version goes like this: I close my eyes (or sometimes not) and, taking a deep breath, I visualize a warm, gentle stream of water pouring over my head, flowing down my spine, and running softly over my body. As the warm, soothing water runs over me, spilling onto the floor, I visualize my stress being washed away. This "mini" mental escape is very effective, and I highly recommend it. (But not when you're driving, operating large equipment, or need to use the bathroom!)

Putting It into Practice

The first thing you'll need to do is pick your destination. You could try the beach, like I chose, or maybe a wooded area, the mountains, or a spot by a stream. Then picture the area in your mind's eye, focusing on a few of your favorite features, such as the sunshine on the water, the wind rustling through the leaves, or the sun setting over distant mountains. Make a mental checklist of these "vacation" highlights to help you find your way there again during your next stressful time of need.

Once you've chosen your mental vacation spot and familiarized yourself with the visualization details, you've got to work on getting yourself there despite any stress you may be feeling. Begin by closing your eyes and reviewing your visualization checklist. Breathe in and out, gently, three times until your mental vacation movie starts playing in your own personal mental theater. Remember to breathe slowly, in and out, as you focus on the details of your movie.

Over time, this exercise will become easier; you'll be able to hop to your mental vacation spot with no trouble, and you will quickly be able to achieve a sense of peace.

six

Journaling

It was a pink diary with a gold key attached to its lock by a silky pastel-pink ribbon. Though a strange place to keep the key for a lock, that's where I kept it. I remember hiding the diary under my mattress and fiercely guarding freshly inked entries revealing the latest objects of my affection. I was nine, and the little pink diary, a gift from Santa Claus, became a trusted friend—a place to share the unshareable.

Even if you didn't have a diary of your own when you were young, you're probably acquainted with the concept of journaling—keeping a written record of your daily life documenting your thoughts, feelings, desires, or interpretations of your life's experiences. What I'd like to offer you, however, is journaling with a little twist—an adult version of the little pink diary. And here's why: control, control, and control!

When Mark and I were in the family-creating mode, our relationship began to shift from romance to mechanics. He became, above all else, the sperm supplier. How quickly we fall from love-making to the pure mechanics of baby-making. I began to hear that old song by the Righteous Brothers, "You've Lost That Loving Feeling," play over and over in my head.

So what does this have to do with a diary?

The goal of journaling is to purge yourself of your daily stressors and emotional thoughts by pouring them out onto the page. Just getting them out of your head and down your arm onto paper will give you a tremendous sense of power and control. Just like your scheduled lamenting time (Strategy Four), journaling releases your "mental toxins." In a sense, your personal journal is a nonjudgmental reflection of your life, bearing witness to your day and providing a safe place for uninhibited release.

Think of journaling as documenting your thoughts and activities of the day for history's sake. Whether you're jotting down your day's activities or venting about an incident that's weighing on your mind, putting things on paper has a way of lessening your burdens and fine-tuning your perspectives. It's a great way to stay sane while trying to make a baby.

At this point some of you might be thinking that this all sounds pretty elementary—and you might be correct. But here's the twist. *I want you to write down your love story.*

Each individual in a couple interprets the baby-creating experience differently, and, because of those differences, it can be easy to "lose that loving feeling." From my experience, it is critical to have direct access to why we're with who we're with, what made us fall head-over-heels in love with that person, and why we committed our-selves to a life with that person. One day when Mark and I were at odds—when the "ugly-marriage" bug began to bite and I interpreted his behavior as unloving, cold, and disinterested—before I went for his jugular, I realized that I wanted a reminder of why I was in love with this person. That night, in my journal, I wrote down our love story. My anger at Mark softened, and I became more rational about the argument we'd had. From then on, whenever things got tense, or our lovemaking became too mechanical, I would reread our history. By doing that, I connected to the "loving feeling" and was able to address my feelings in a controlled manner.

Putting It into Practice

You may already be a convert to journaling for your own personal growth. If you are, I encourage you to start a new journal to record just your experiences as you try to become parents. When you finally achieve your goal—and you will!—you'll be able to store this journal away as a separate chapter in your life.

If you're new to journaling, I think you'll find it—and this exercise in particular—very helpful.

- Determine what you will be using for your journal: a notebook, loose-leaf paper in a binder, a store-bought journal, even a real diary, complete with lock and key. You might want to purchase a special pen to use just for this journal.

- Find a time when you'll be undisturbed and can write in peace.

- Open your new journal to the fresh first page. In the upper right-hand corner, write the date that you met your partner. Not today's date, but the date your relationship began, the date you first met this person who you now may be viewing as a sperm- or egg-making machine.

* Then begin to fill the page with the sights, sounds, smells, and feelings of that meeting.

* When you're finished with that, write down five reasons why you fell in love with him or her.

* As you and your partner continue in your quest to have a baby, refer to your love story again and again. Trust me—this really works. Your documentation of your meeting, and its significance to you, is the key to accessing those loving feelings again.

It is said that on average it takes twenty-one days to create a habit. I ask that you commit to journaling for at least that amount of time and feel the power and reap the benefits!

seven

The Gratitude List

Mark and I arrived at our seminar just in the nick of time. We were scheduled to present our "Strategies to Save your Sanity and Relationship While Trying to Have a Baby" seminar to a group of patients from the same medical practice. Mark took a seat in the front row and I addressed the group.

"Good evening, my name is Kristen Magnacca, and it's a pleasure to be here this evening. I'd like to start with one of my most favorite quotes, from Oliver Wendell Holmes: 'Sometimes a moment's insight is worth a lifetime's experience.'

"Tonight my husband, Mark, and I are going to share some of our insights and strategies for saving your sanity and keeping your relationship in balance while creating your family. You could say Mark and I are 'out of the closet' with our fertility challenges and how they affected us both individually and as a couple. Our quest to have a baby brought us to a place so far from the bedroom that we weren't sure if our relationship would survive.

"By day, Mark and I were working with companies to help them communicate more effectively, deal with change, and gain a sense of control over their company's mission and vision; at night, we discarded what we knew worked so well in our business lives, came home, and unknowingly sabotaged our personal lives. We both wanted a baby—that was one of the only things we knew for sure. But the manner in which we handled the process was drastically different. That's when we got into trouble."

As I spoke to the group, I became distracted by a woman sitting in the front row with her husband. The suit she wore was wrinkled from a long day's work and her eyes looked tired as she tilted to one side. Her dark hair, hovering around her chin, barely masked tears that gently fell as she listened to my story.

I continued, "Mark and I tried for months to conceive a child and were unsuccessful. We were doing what we were supposed to at the appropriate time and failing. It was our first crisis as a couple, and we weren't prepared for our different approaches. Then we finally heard the words that every couple longs for—'You're pregnant!'—and we reveled in the intense joy that those words carried. Then the world came crashing in: We lost this baby because the pregnancy was ectopic. We almost lost our marriage as well."

The woman's shoulders began to shake; tears were streaming down her face as she reached for another Kleenex.

I'm usually pretty composed when speaking publicly, but with this window into her sadness I began to feel myself losing it. Out of my mouth popped, "We're going to take a bathroom break, and when we get back we're going to get moving onto some exercises." I barely got the words out as I was walking to the back of the room. Once the group broke up, I turned to the wall and began to cry. My friend and staunch supporter, Roseann, who was helping facilitate that evening's seminar, was suddenly at my side.

"What's wrong with you? Are you crying?" she asked.

"There's a woman sitting in the front row who's sobbing. I could just feel her sadness and began to lose it myself."

I was very surprised at my reaction to this woman. I had presented to similar groups across the country and there were numerous occasions when attendees became emotional, yet I wasn't affected. This time was different. The woman's sorrow was so intense that I could feel her sadness and pain.

Mark appeared at my side and told me he'd felt it, too. Then he swung into his "Mr. Fix-It" mode. "We have to get going again, so let's regroup here for a moment, then start back up. I'll take over for the first exercise and then you jump in," he said.

There we had it—a recovery plan.

Mark swung into gear, bringing the group through the first exercise and then introducing the journaling strategy and the complementing strategy of a Gratitude List.

"Kristen is going to take over again and explain the concept of a Gratitude List," he announced. As Mark took my seat, I assumed his spot at the front of the room.

"I remember the day I implemented the Gratitude List," I began. "It was one of those days when I was so whiny I could barely stand myself. I knew I needed to do something different, so I called a friend who works as a family therapist, and what he said to me was like a slap across the face. He said, 'I can't believe what I'm hearing from you, Kristen! Absolutely no gratitude?! You have gone from a person whose glass was half-full to a half-empty kind of person. Where is your gratitude?' he asked me.

"He really upset me! I was thinking, 'Where did he get off?' And then I heard what he was saying: I was so focused on what I *didn't* have—a baby—that I totally lost focus on what I *did* have. The everyday, life-enhancing things—my husband bringing me that first cup of coffee in the morning, a clean towel after my shower, a completed 'to do' list at the end of a workday, a dinner out and a chocolate chip cookie, a full tank of gas—they all meant nothing to me because I was childless.

"So that night, after I purged the emotions of our conversation onto the page, something clicked. At the end of my journal entry I jotted down a list of six things I felt grateful for. From then on, when I began to feel the emotion of 'lack' starting to drive my mental bus, I focused on my list. I focused on the *positive* things I have to be grateful for. Saying it over and over again, it became my mantra; in a singsong inner voice I repeated and repeated my Gratitude List and drifted off to sleep. It was the first good night's sleep I'd had in about six months," I concluded.

The first-row woman let go of one last sob, and then her face lit up.

At that point, I directed the group to take the next few minutes and jot down five or six things that they were grateful for. I pushed the button for some quiet background music and turned around to see the audience working away. We made eye contact for the first time, the front-row woman and I, and she winked at me. I smiled back.

It was hectic at the close of the seminar as both Mark and I engaged in conversation with a few of the couples. I wanted to have a personal conversation with the woman in the front row and offer some help, but she was gone.

About three weeks later, I received an e-mail in my inbox from a name I didn't recognize. It began with "*You might not remember me but I attended one of your seminars that you gave about three weeks ago. I sat in the front row with my husband."*

It was the front-row woman, who had been on my mind since the seminar.

"The night of your seminar, I was so upset because we had just made the decision to start artificial insemination. I wanted to let you know that at first I didn't try your strategy about gratitude. You see, I have been experiencing insomnia for a while now and feeling totally overwhelmed around our attempts to conceive. Then I tried it, and for two weeks now I have been adding what I am grateful for to the end of my journal, and I say them over and over. I've been able to sleep for two weeks now and use the list sometimes during the day, too. I just wanted to say thank you."

That night I listed her e-mail as one of things I was grateful for that day. Talk about karma!

Putting It into Practice

As I shared with you in this story, the Gratitude List is a complement to the act of journaling. At the end of your nightly journal entry, write down, in list form, five or six things that you're grateful for. You may find that on particularly rough days, it's hard to come up with at least five things. But I encourage you to push yourself. You can do it—and it's worth your effort.

The second half of the strategy is to use the list as a mantra to refocus your thoughts on what you do have in your life, not what it's lacking.

Make your cup half-full instead of half-empty.

Think Abundance

I was driving in a bit of a hurry. I got stuck at a red light and drummed my fingers on the steering wheel. "Come on, come *on*," I urged under my breath.

The light turned green; being first in line, I gunned the accelerator. Driving a little faster than the speed limit, I was making good time. Then, up ahead of me in the distance, I saw a car, a Buick Park Avenue. It was the same model my mom bought upon her retirement, and ever since my family has referred to it as the "standard issue" for retirees. This particular Buick was moving at a quarter of the posted speed limit. I could have run faster.

Braking, I slowed to a snail's pace behind the Buick, and realized that the elderly man behind the wheel was wearing a hat. Another running joke in my family is to beware of old men driving—especially those wearing hats! Slow as molasses.

I was so irritated my stomach churned, and I beeped my horn. My behavior was surprising; I was completely out of control and unable to manage my state of mind.

Finally I passed him and shot him one of those "you shouldn't be driving!" looks.

When I got to my destination, I was feeling quite disappointed in myself. At that point in my life, disappointment had become the common theme. There was disappointment in our marriage because of miscommunication, disappointment with our inability to conceive a child, and disappointment in my management of the whole situation. The disappointment spilled over into all aspects of my life and, on that day, it was driving. And through my disappointment-tinted glasses, the man in the hat was an annoyance, as opposed to an angel.

My normal life philosophy is that everything happens for a reason. Although I may not be totally conscious of the reason from the start, in my experience the universe has a way of revealing the answer eventually. Looked at in this light, even the old man in the hat was there for a reason.

Which brings us to Strategy Eight: Think Abundance. Similar in concept to the Gratitude List, Thinking Abundance will help you maintain a positive flow of energy in your body.

The key lies in what I call the "three A's": Awareness, Acceptance, and, finally, Abundance. Let's put the three A's into action by revisiting my encounter with the man in the hat. This will demonstrate how they all connect to my philosophy that everything happens for a reason.

I was driving in a bit of a hurry. I got stuck at a red light and drummed my fingers on the steering wheel. "Come on, come *on*," I urged under my breath.

The light turned green; being first in line, I gunned the accelerator. Driving a little faster than the speed limit, I was making good time. Then, up ahead of me in the distance, I saw a car, a Buick Park

Avenue. It was the same model my mom bought upon her retirement, and ever since my family has referred to it as the "standard issue" for retirees. This particular Buick was moving at a quarter of the posted speed limit. I could have run faster.

Braking, I slowed to a snail's pace behind the Buick, and realized that the elderly man behind the wheel was wearing a hat. It's a running joke in my family to beware of old men driving—especially those wearing hats! Slow as molasses.

I was so irritated my stomach churned, and I beeped my horn. When I went to beep it again, though, I paused.

I pulled myself out of my "intense-driver" mode and became fully aware of the situation I was in and my present surroundings. I asked myself: Why did the universe send the man in the hat to me? (*Awareness*)

Forcing back the instinct to beep again and zoom past the guy, I looked at my watch, accepting that I was going to be a few minutes late. I reached for my cell phone and called the person I was supposed to meet to tell him I was running about five minutes behind schedule, which was fine with him. (*Acceptance*)

Then I got the sense I was being slowed down for a reason; perhaps an accident was waiting for me further down the road if I kept up my current hurried pace. Or was it possible I was supposed to meet someone outside the building where my appointment was scheduled who I would have missed if I didn't slow down? Maybe the lesson I was supposed to learn from the man in the hat was tolerance or, for God's sake, patience. Patience with the unexpected setbacks in life, and patience with the process of conception. (*Abundance*)

Having utilized Awareness first, Acceptance then flowed with ease. Accepting my current situation enabled me to manage it while maintaining balance. In the few seconds it took to call and let my colleague know I was running a little behind, my body relaxed, and I arrived safely, and calm.

Which leads us to Abundance. At this point, I was free to feel grateful for my understanding and patience, and trust that the universe was giving me the tools from which to learn. I began to focus on the abundance in my life, on what I *had*, instead of what I thought I *didn't* have—enough time.

Webster's Dictionary defines abundance as "a more than plentiful quantity of something" or "a lifestyle with more than adequate material provisions" or "a fullness of spirit that overflows." For me, Abundance was the most important of the three A's.

But after so many attempts at creating our family, I could not see me fitting into any of Webster's definitions. I remember the debilitating feelings that would rush over me whenever I saw a pregnant woman. The sight of a round, full belly would send me into an emotional fit of "lack," and I would literally have to remove myself from the woman's presence. Many a time I had to cut an outing short after seeing a baby or a pregnant woman, and head home early, feeling upset, disappointed, and angry over the fact we were childless. My behavior resembled an anxiety disorder stemming from the fear of seeing a baby or pregnant woman.

Then Mark and I attended a seminar given by fertility expert Dr. Ali Domar, in which she taught us the concept of "Mindfulness." Dr. Domar led the group in an exercise in how to stay "in the moment" by slowly eating a piece of chocolate and calling on all of our five senses while we did so.

At first I felt a little silly, slowly and carefully unwrapping the Hershey's Kiss, feeling the aluminum foil between my fingers, smelling the first whiff of chocolate escape into the air. I examined the Kiss, then took one small bite, allowing the chocolate to melt slowly instead of popping the whole thing in my mouth and devouring it within seconds.

As usual, Mark's appetite took over; his chocolate Kiss was history before I even had mine unwrapped. His idea of Mindfulness— eating the whole thing in one bite—is a perfect example of how hard it is to train yourself to dwell in the moment. But, with some practice, we both got it down, bringing us back to a place of Abundance, a place where I could control my anxiety around pregnant women by focusing on the positive currents surrounding me.

Mindfulness gave me the tools to refocus and look for what I had—my Abundance. Instead of spoiling a whole evening by obsessing over the pregnant woman or the beautiful baby, I tuned my brain to the positive details, listing them in my head: "Here I am, out with Mark, the man I love, in a wonderful restaurant. I don't have to cook, and someone else will serve me, clean up after me, and bring me dessert. This is exactly what I needed."

Putting It into Practice

1. Create the habit of being aware. Awareness, by definition, is understanding that something exists because you notice it or realize that it is happening. Notice what's going on around you. Whether it's a positive or a negative situation, ask yourself what the reason for its occurrence could be. Here are some sample internal questions that you can use: Why is this situation being presented to me? How else could this problem be solved? What possibilities does this circumstance bring with it?

2. Practice Acceptance. The universe has a plan, on its own time-line, not ours, and it's your acceptance of this plan or situation that can unblock your energy.

3. Think Abundance. Practicing Awareness and Acceptance frees you to focus on abundance, gratitude, understanding, and patience, and will foster a sense of trust that the universe is providing you experiences or tools for you to learn from. When you rejoice in what you have, and turn your thoughts away from what you don't have, you're releasing a flow of energy that is creative rather than unproductive. Think back to the two driving scenarios I related earlier. Do you see yourself in the first driving example or the second? It's a struggle to be the person in the second scenario focusing on Abundance—what we have—instead of what we think we don't have. But how can that sense of spirit be created and sustained while dealing with such constant negative emotion? Practice, practice, and practice again making the choice to create a lifestyle that has a fullness of spirit that will overflow into the creation of your family.

A Fertility Log

As I opened the blue-covered notebook, my internal voice mimicked Captain Kirk of the *Starship Enterprise*: "Mission Log, my follicle size today is 9." The log was a daily journal of the changes in my bodily signs, hormonal levels, and follicle size while I progressed through a cycle of artificial insemination. It made me feel as though I were the commander of the *Starship Kristen*, carefully keeping a log of what my body was experiencing and where it might go on its intergalactic journey.

In hindsight, I wish I had kept a log from the beginning, when we first started counting the days of my monthly cycle, then using a basal thermometer to record my daily temperature, and finally an ovulation predictor before entering the world of assisted reproductive technology. A self-contained log listing our initial attempts at conceiving would have armed me with information for discussion with my medical team while also documenting my body's cycles.

When I purchased a "pee-on-the-stick" ovulation monitor, I thought it was going to be a one-time experience. Yet I ended up using it for several months, never writing down my daily results. After six or seven months without the benefits of the written log, I began to regret my failure to document, for I never really knew if my body was behaving regularly.

I would say to myself, "I think I got two bars, which indicated the beginning of ovulation on the predictor machine last month on day ten. Now it's day eleven and I'm not ovulating. This would send me into a panic, thinking that my body wasn't working correctly and I wasn't going to ovulate, or that I was premenopausal. All these negative feelings could have been avoided had I just documented my cycles.

Once I did begin keeping a Fertility Log, it became my best friend. Not only did it provide me with another concrete example of our progress on our mystifying journey to parenthood, but it also contained the history of our procreation, offering me great hope by showing me that my body *was* changing during the cycle and creating an environment for a baby.

When Mark and I had progressed to assisted reproductive technology, using intrauterine insemination, I was required each morning to sign in at the clinic to secure my place in the blood drawing line. Upon doing so, I would write my telephone number and then, in capital letters, "LEAVE NUMBERS PLEASE." Each evening, the nurse would call with my nightly instructions and she would also tell me my hormone levels and follicle size. I would carefully write the information down in the log, which gave me an incredible sense of my accomplishment. My arms ached to be holding our child. It was the "mission" of all our efforts. But in the interim, we would celebrate the growth of my follicles that were bringing us to the point of insemination.

When I heard my daily numbers, I would do a little follicle dance! "Go Kristen! Go Kristen! It might be your baby's birthday!" I would chant to myself. As crazy as it sounds, it helped. I was focusing on creating and working toward providing the best possible baby-making environment, and this simple log chronicled my efforts.

Putting It into Practice

Whether you're counting days, using natural signs (such as vaginal mucus changes), recording your basal temperature, or are currently in a treatment cycle, it's important to keep all of your information in its own special book. Centralizing your observations and records will provide insights into your cycles, show you your bodily rhythms, and give you a sense of control.

Just like you did for your personal thought journal, choose the medium and location for your Fertility Log that work best for you. I used a notebook and left it by the phone. That was appropriate for Mark and me, but you do what's most convenient for you.

There's another important part of the log: Celebrate small victories. You certainly don't have to be as outrageous as I was, with my follicle dance and rah-rah chanting, but celebrating small victories is a must. You could have a piece of cake or paint your toenails blue, or purchase your husband or partner an appropriate surprise gift (maybe some boxer shorts?).

In our experience, celebrating during the positive moments helps to make the unbearable moments more bearable.

II

Communicating as One

Unlock Your Partner's Communication Strategy

*I*t was a surprise. I was told to be dressed up and ready to go at 6:00 PM. Right on schedule, we hopped into the car and headed toward Providence, Rhode Island.

"So, where are we going? Will you tell me now?" I asked Mark.

"We're going to see *RENT!*" he announced.

I was thrilled! I had been trying to see the play for over a year and, for one reason or another, it hadn't ever worked out.

After we arrived at the theater and took our seats, the lights blinked and the audience hushed in anticipation as the curtain rose. The actors began singing out their stories, and I sat perfectly still, basking in the music that filled the air.

"What are they talking about?" Mark whispered, interrupting my basking in the moment of the play.

I quickly brought him up to speed, feeling as though I were interpreting a foreign language for him. He nodded his understanding, and I gratefully turned my attention back to the stage, hoping he wouldn't be requiring any more of my translating services.

Yet, as the music changed tempo and the plot thickened, I received another nudge from my husband.

"What's happening now?" Mark was the only one breaking the silence of the audience.

"What's wrong with you? Aren't you listening?" I asked.

After several more interruptions, I finally tuned him out, losing myself in the play. But moments later, when I realized that the nudging and questions had stopped altogether, I glanced Mark's way and found him sound asleep, head back, mouth open.

Quickly suppressing a twinge of embarrassment, I accepted his silence and left him to his slumber, enjoying the play by myself.

Mark has an inability to understand words to songs. Always has, always will. He marvels at the fact that I can sing a song word-for-word and accuses me of making up the lyrics. Frank Sinatra is Mark's favorite, but Ol' Blue Eyes would be rolling over in his grave if he knew how dreadfully Mark butchers his lyrics.

The differences in our communication abilities don't end with our lyric-translating skills. It was when Mark and I first started using the "L" word that we began to realize the differences in our communication strategies. I would tell Mark that I loved him every time we finished a telephone conversation and spontaneously when we were together. One day, however, he said to me, "Boy, you need to hear that a lot." Not necessarily music to my ears! This comment triggered an ugly banter that started something like this:

"Well, don't worry, buddy, you're not gonna hear that again from me if it's so bothersome."

The fight-train had left the station and was chugging its way down ugly track Number 1 until Mark apologized and shared with me a test he had taken that would help us communicate more effectively. The questions in this test helped us pin down the differences in our communication strategies so that we could adjust to each other's individual needs and avoid future misunderstandings.

Every brain is wired uniquely. Our personalities, how we talk and communicate, and our interpretation of the world boil down to neural connections in our brains, and it is these connections that also determine how you and your partner communicate and connect. Strategy Eleven will teach you how to unlock your partner's unique communication strategy.

To preface how this strategy works, remember that if you are right-handed it doesn't mean that you never use your left hand. Likewise, if you score highest on the visual checklist it doesn't mean that you're not a feeling or auditory person. It just indicates that your preferred strategy for interpreting information is visual. In fact, some people are equally balanced between the three modalities. Most people, though, have one dominant style.

The Visuals: These are people whose filter is dominated by their sight. They're usually well groomed and very organized around the house and with their personal items. These people are not clutter bugs. When they speak, they often use words such as "clearly," and phrases like, "I see what you're saying," or "I'm in a fog."

The Auditories: Then there are the "auditory" people, who love to listen to music, seem to have bionic ears that can hear through walls, and possess the ability to recall conversations word-for-word. Their language patterns consist of phrases such as, "I hear what you're saying," and "That doesn't ring a bell." They're not very concerned with how things look and might appear disorganized.

The Kinesthetics: The last group is people who are "kinesthetic," or wired for feeling. Men who are kinesthetic often wear a beard that they stroke while talking. Their vocabulary consists of phrases like, "That doesn't feel right to me," or instead of saying, "I *think* you are keeping something from me," they will say, "I *feel* like you are keeping something from me." You'll notice that they take a longer than normal time to respond to questions because they are assessing their feelings about the event or issue. They seem to talk and move a little more slowly than others.

As evident in my role as Mark's translator of lyrics and my fondness for using the "L" word, I'm a hearing-oriented, or "auditory" person. I interpret words with a strong auditory sense. Mark, on the other hand, has a strong feeling sense. He's kinesthetic, which is why I've learned to touch his arm when I want to speak with him. I am more apt to lose his attention if I don't.

Mark and I have adapted an "Information Preference Checklist" created by marketing strategist Dr. Donald Moine. This assessment tool is from his book *Modern Persuasion Strategies*. We use this checklist in our seminars to help couples learn about each other's individual communication preferences. You'll find this assessment tool in the *Putting It into Practice* section of this chapter. But to get a better feel for how the test works and what it has to offer, let's look at the results of one particular couple who attended one of our seminars.

This couple's results revealed that the husband was feeling-oriented, whereas his wife was sight-oriented. He was wearing a soft sweater and sat very relaxed in his chair; she wore her hair short and was dressed very neatly in a turtleneck and slacks. As he melted into the chair, his breathing was slow and paced, while his wife's was quick and rapid. He took time to digest ideas that we were discussing and, when adding to the conversation, she finished his sentences because her timing was quicker. She accessed her association to what was happening visually, while her husband felt his way through the exchange.

When Mark asked what attracted him to his wife, he said, "She has the ability to come into a room and quickly make things happen."

He frequently reached over and touched her hand. When Mark asked what attracted her to her husband, she responded, "He adds stability to my life and is thoughtful about his decision-making." Then Mark asked if those same qualities are frustrating at times, and, as the whole group laughed, it was agreed upon that what made us fall in love with our partners can also be a great source of conflict.

"Would you say that sometimes you have to wait for your husband to respond or take action?" Mark asked the woman.

"Yes, most definitely," she replied.

"How does that make you feel?" Mark inquired.

"Well, I've gotten used to it, but it can be frustrating at times." As she spoke, her husband reached over and rubbed her back. "But seeing this in black and white makes me realize the difference."

Moving on to demonstrate how this information can help in communication, Mark made the following suggestion. First he addressed the wife:

"You might want to slow your speech down when you talk to your husband and reach over and touch his hand or arm. Kristen does this when she wants me to stay focused, fulfilling the feeling part of me first and then saying what needs to be communicated."

To the husband, Mark made the following suggestions: "Your wife is a visual person and you might want to use language that compliments this style, such as 'I can see what you're saying,' and 'It's clear to me now.' The written word is a great way to communicate with your wife. Taking a moment to write down bullet points before engaging in a serious discussion would work wonderfully.

"Remember," Mark continued, "We each have a dominant way of communicating, but it's not the *only* way we can communicate. Keeping this in mind can help avoid miscommunication and misunderstandings."

Putting It into Practice

To discover into which communication category you and your partner fall, complete the checklists below.

Read each statement under the three categories and check the ones that relate to you.

At the end of each section add up the number of items that you checked, putting the total on the line provided.

When all three sections are completed, your highest score reveals your most dominant communication strategy.

Visual Orientation

☐ On an evening when I don't have anything else to do, I like to watch TV.

☐ I use visual images to remember names.

☐ I like to read books and magazines.

☐ I prefer to get written instructions from my boss rather than oral ones.

☐ I write lists to myself of things I have to do.

☐ I follow recipes closely when I am cooking.

☐ I can easily put together models and toys if I have written instructions.

☐ When it comes to playing games, I prefer word games like Scrabble or Password.

☐ I am very concerned about the way I look.

☐ I like to go to art exhibits and museum displays.

☐ I keep a diary or a written record of what I have been doing.

☐ I often admire the photographs and artwork used in advertisements.

☐ I review for a test by writing down a summary of all pertinent points.

□   I can find my way around a new city easily if I have a map.

□   I like to keep my house very neat.

□   I see two or more films each month.

□   I think less highly of a person if he or she does not dress nicely.

□   I like to watch people.

□   I always get scratches and dents repaired quickly on my car.

□   I think fresh flowers really brighten up a home or office.

____   **Total Score for Visual Orientation**

Auditory Orientation

□   On an evening when I don't have anything else to do, I like to listen to music.

□   To remember someone's name, I will repeat it to myself over and over again.

□   I enjoy long conversations.

□   I prefer having my boss explain something to me rather than write a memo.

□   I like talk shows and interview shows on radio and television.

□   I use rhyming words to help me remember things.

□   I am a good listener.

□   I prefer to keep up with the news by listening to the radio rather than by reading.

□   I talk to myself a lot.

□   I prefer to listen to a cassette tape of some material rather than to read it.

□   I feel bad when my car sounds funny (has knocks, pings, etc.).

□   I can tell a lot about a person by the sound of his or her voice.

□   I buy a lot of CDs and prerecorded tapes.

□   I review for a test by reading my notes aloud or by talking with other people.

□   I would rather give a talk than write a paper on the same topic.

□   I enjoy going to concerts and musical events.

□   People sometimes accuse me of talking too much.

☐ When I am in a strange city, I like to stop at a gas station to get directions.

☐ I talk to my dog or cat.

☐ I talk aloud to myself when I'm solving a math problem.

____ **Total Score for Auditory Orientation**

Kinesthetic (Feeling-Movement-Touch) Orientation

☐ I like to exercise.

☐ When I am blindfolded, I can distinguish items by touch.

☐ When there is music on, I can't help but tap my feet.

☐ I am an outdoors person.

☐ I am well coordinated.

☐ I have a tendency to gain weight.

☐ I buy some clothes because I like the way the material feels.

☐ I like to pet animals.

☐ I touch people when I am talking with them.

☐ When I was learning to type, I learned the touch system easily.

☐ I was held and touched a lot when I was a child.

☐ I enjoy playing sports more than watching them.

☐ I like taking a hot bath at the end of a day.

☐ I really enjoy getting massages.

☐ I am a good dancer.

☐ I belong to a gym or health spa.

☐ I like to get up and stretch frequently.

☐ I can tell a lot about a person by the way he or she shakes hands.

☐ If I've had a bad day, my body gets very tense.

☐ I enjoy crafts, handiworks, and/or building things.

____ **Total Score for Kinesthetic Orientation**

[Adapted from "Information Preference Checklist" on pp. 49–51 from Modern Persuasion Strategies: The Hidden Advantage in Selling, by Donald J. Moine. Dr. Moine (www.drmoine.com), is a pioneer in applying neurolinguistic programming to regular life.]

Knowing how your partner communicates most effectively can and will improve the process. It's like knowing that your partner loves green beans for dinner and making them as often as possible.

Find his or her favorite communication style and serve that baby up!

eleven

The Association Game

Several years ago, on our way to give the keynote address at an infertility symposium in New Hampshire, Mark and I stopped at an Italian restaurant for a warm meal and a quick prep session for our upcoming speech on expectations.

"I've color-coded the sheet; you're blue," I said, sliding a colorful sheet of paper across the table to Mark. This color-coded, grid-like diagram that we typically use to organize our speeches is called a mind map, and it breaks down the seminar or speech into blocks. Each block is clearly labeled to indicate who will be speaking and what topics will be covered. This helps us keep the presentation flowing and organized.

Mark chewed on crusty Italian bread, crumbs falling on the sheet, while he reviewed his portion.

"Good, you put me down for the associations exercise; that's always a good one. Hey, we haven't done that in months. We should do it now as a refresher," he noted.

"Okay, what word do you want to use?" I asked.

"Infertility."

For the next few moments we sat across from each other with our heads bent over our papers, candles providing our reading light.

"Done," I said.

"Me too. You go first," Mark said.

When I finished reading my list of ten words and Mark read off his, we had only two common words between us. Two little words. After five years of presenting and sharing our strategy, we still brought our own unique interpretations to our situation. My ten words were very emotional: *sadness, pain, tired, misunderstanding,* and *longing* were a few. Mark's words were very clinical in nature: *procedure, time-consuming, doctors, clinic, test,* and *blood.* We both had *pain* and *sadness.*

"I can't believe we only have two words in common!" Mark said. "What is that all about? You know, we're still miles apart on this issue and will probably always be, but what's so important about this exercise is that it shows how it really is about each person's own interpretation."

"Yes, and it's really okay that you're wrong about your interpretations and I'm not," I informed Mark. We both laughed.

I continued, "No really, it's important that we don't start a riot between the partners at the seminar tomorrow. We need to emphasize that the purpose of this exercise is not to show the great divide between them, but to highlight where each person is in the process and what it all means to them personally."

"I totally agree, it's not that you still have such strong emotional associations to the word that is so important, but that *knowing* you do helps me to understand how you feel about the situation," Mark added.

"Pretty powerful and cool stuff," I said with a smile.

The next morning, Mark and I were in the middle of presenting our keynote address and arrived at the Association Game square of the mind map. Mark jumped in to do the section.

"Right now we're all sitting in the same room, listening to a presentation," he began. "But we are all noticing totally different things. You might be distracted by the hum of the overhead fan, or the flicker of the light in the back of the room. Some of us might be noticing the temperature, or the fact that I'm pacing.

"There are a hundred of us in this room, and we are all taking in different stimuli that give this experience meaning to us. We've all heard how two people witnessing an accident can give completely different accounts of what they saw. How does that happen?

"It's all about how we filter our world, which then determines what we associate to something. We'd like you to play along with us for a few minutes and do this exercise. Use the paper we left on your seat.

"Quickly write down ten words that you associate with the word 'baby.' Go ahead and get started. When you and your partner have each written ten words, one of you read your list. If you and your partner have the same word on your lists, circle it. So, ready, set, go!"

The room fell quiet and the soft music overhead filled in the silence.

After a few minutes passed and the murmuring between couples had fallen off, Mark again addressed the audience.

"Okay, how many people had ten for ten?" He waited a few seconds, and no one raised his or her hand.

"Okay, how many couples had nine, eight, or seven?" Again no hands in the air.

"Okay, six, five, four, or three?" Moving himself around the room, Mark noticed a hand!

"Great, how many words in common?" he asked.

"Three," the male partner answered with pride.

"Wow, good for you guys, will you share what they were?" Mark asked.

"Parents, pain, and sadness," the man answered again.

"Did anyone else have those three on their paper?" Mark addressed the whole audience.

"How about two, one, or no words in common?" The majority of the hands in the audience went up.

While this exchange was building, I was watching the interaction between a couple sitting to Mark's left. The woman was obviously upset with her husband and I was waiting for the appropriate time to jump in to Mark's discussion and direct my attention to them.

"To be honest with you, we expected the outcome of this exercise to be one or none, and I'll tell you why this is important—"

Before Mark could finish I jumped in.

"I have to tell you what happened to Mark and me last night at dinner," I blurted out. "Here we are, years into our baby-creating journey, living what we preach, so to speak, and we sat down to do this exercise ourselves. We had two words alike! Yes, two little words! I had a flash of anger directed at Mark because he wasn't on the same wavelength as me and, to me, his associations were way out in left field. At least that's how I interpreted them at first. His were all wrong!

"But then I remembered the true purpose of this exercise. The true purpose is to show where the other person is in the experience, to expose his or her interpretation of events so that, as a couple, you can come to an understanding about feelings, hopes, and desires."

I walked over to the couple and addressed the woman, who was still upset. "May I ask you how many words you had in common?"

The woman snapped back, "None."

"Well, when Mark and I did this exercise for the first time we had none in common, too, and it just added to my frustration," I said. "So here's what we did, we started to talk about the words on the paper and asked each other why they wrote them and what they meant. After we did that, I felt connected to Mark, more than I had in a long time. It was an eye-opening exercise because it gave Mark an opportunity to share his feelings with me, and mine with him—without him trying to fix anything. You know how the male brain can swing into Mr. Fix-It mode."

She laughed and touched her husband's hand.

"So, in a way, having no words in common was the best possible outcome for us and being losers at the Association Game was a gift to our marriage!" I exclaimed.

"Once again, Kristen throws me under the bus!" Mark chimed in.

"All for a good cause, dear!"

Putting It into Practice

For the first round of the Association Game, use the word "baby."

- ❀ Write down ten words that pop into your head when you hear the word "baby."
- ❀ Pick one partner to read his or her list, circling the words that you both have in common as the words are being read.
- ❀ Add up the number of circled words.
- ❀ Begin discussing the words. You can start with the words that you both have in common or with the ones that aren't

circled. In order to better understand your partner's perception, start with the question, "Why did you put that word on
your list?"

✿ Hug and kiss at the end of the exercise. (This is a must!)

This exercise is immeasurably helpful for opening lines of communication and coming to a sense of understanding with your partner.
You can also use it when you find yourself at an impasse (a nice way
of saying "argument"). Choose a word that describes the conflict
point and work from there.

Understanding what is associated with any given circumstance
will help to weave the fabric of your marriage together, more tightly
and more securely than before!

twelve

Pain vs. Pleasure

*T*he silence in the house was deafening. Mark was hidden away in his home office and I was in mine. We were in the midst of a marital discussion gone wrong. For the life of me, I could not figure out how we had taken such a terrible turn to heated words and angry gestures.

After hours of avoiding each other, we accidentally met in the hallway heading for the kitchen.

"Want a hug?" Mark came at me, arms extended.

"No, hug *this!*" I snapped, and stuck out my tongue. Mark followed me into the bathroom, spun me around, and looked into my eyes. Suddenly, we both began to laugh at our childish behavior.

A friend who's a family therapist shared with us once that it's not the heated marital discussion itself that hurts a marriage; the real damage is done by the amount of time it takes to recover from it. Luckily for us, this one was brief, and we were able to break the downward spiral with laughter.

How did we get here, though? We were both on the same sheet of music—we had our Fertility Game Plan, we did the Association Game, and we knew where the other stood regarding having a baby. We were working through this period of transition, yet still hit a huge marital speed bump when deciding our next step toward becoming parents.

This was the conflict: I wanted to continue for a few more months on the alternative methods path before reentering the world of assisted reproductive technology (ART) and beginning a cycle of in vitro fertilization. Mark, on the other hand, felt as though we were wasting time with the alternative therapies. He thought we could get to our family quicker through IVF. We both wanted the same outcome, but had different views about how to get there.

One of the things we discovered about each other through all of this is that we both have different motivational, or decision-making strategies. Just as our brains are wired to interpret information through vision, hearing, or feeling, our brains are wired for certain patterns in decision-making as well.

Studies have shown that people are motivated either to move away from pain or to move toward pleasure. Recognizing which strategy you use and which one your partner uses can help you avoid marital hot spots.

I'm a move-away-from-pain kind of gal and Mark is a move-toward-pleasure kind of guy. Enter the "marital discussion gone wrong" regarding the timing of our next step toward being parents.

The pain of childlessness and the very different pain associated with some of the ART techniques were so intense for me that I was doing everything and anything to move away from that type of pain or what I labeled as pain. So I chose ovulation testing, meditation, craniosacral therapy, and acupuncture before attempting the high-tech approach.

Mark was seeking pleasure, and in this instance the pleasure was a child. He was motivated to enter into the high-tech world more quickly because he determined that we would arrive at our outcome, a child, sooner rather than later.

No wonder he viewed my behavior as crazy. I was acting like Goldilocks, trying different alternative methods until I found the perfect fit that would spare me the pain of our situation. As for my interpretation of Mark, I viewed his behavior as callous, cold, and without understanding. Eventually, we both came to understand that each of us was harboring erroneous interpretations of the other.

Here is another example from the repertoire of Kristen and Mark's marriage: Mark needs to say what has been accomplished from our "to do" list in order to motivate himself to complete more, while I list what still needs to be completed to motivate me to keep going. Before we became aware of our differences, his strategy of motivation used to aggravate me to no end because I was focused on completing the list, while he was celebrating what was done! Knowing all of this, I still do get annoyed sometimes at his strategy, but I am able to remind myself why it is important for Mark and I try to view the celebrating in the middle of the list as a break or a gift. It's truly amazing how much can be learned from your partner!

Putting It into Practice

This strategy is so much more than a glass-half-empty person versus a glass-half-full person. It's really about how you're motivated to take action. Why is this important?

It's important because, when compromising with your partner about making a decision, it's helpful to have the right combination to their decision-making lock. Then you can decode the communication and understand how your partner will take action. Failure to acknowledge the fact that people make decisions for different reasons can leave you feeling frustrated, and trying to motivate someone else the way you are motivated can be a colossal waste of time.

Read the statements below and circle the answers that most closely reflect your response.

When exercising, you think:
1. "I have to exercise so that I will not gain weight."
2. "I have to exercise because I like looking fit."

When you think of your car, you think:
3. "I purchased my car because it met my needs."
4. "I purchased my car because it's fun to drive and I love the way it looks."

When ordering a pizza, you say:
5. "I don't want anchovies or onions."
6. "I would like pepperoni and mushrooms."

If you circled 1, 3, and 5, you tend to move away from pain when making a decision. If you circled 2, 4, and 6, you tend to move toward pleasure when making a decision. All of us use both of these strategies for different things, but one strategy tends to dominate.

It's also important to be aware that it's not what the person says as much as the sequence he or she uses when saying it. By this I mean that a person who answers the question by saying first what they don't want typically organizes information in a moving away from pain strategy, whereas the person who first says what they want moves toward pleasure.

Now that you are aware of this information, how can you apply this to the way you communicate with your partner? If you know that your partner's decision-making process involves moving toward pleasure, when you are faced with coming to a mutual decision about a topic, you will benefit from stating your position in a way that focuses on the pleasurable results your method will achieve, as opposed to stating the problem that needs to be addressed. The total opposite applies to a person who moves away from pain—state the problem that needs to be overcome first, then provide a solution.

The "Elevator Speech"™

I **dreaded going to holidays or group functions** when we were in the baby-creating mode because—inevitably—someone would ask THE question.

"So, when are you two going to have a baby?" Aunt Clarice would ask.

This question sent me into a panic. Scanning the room in vain for Mark to come to my rescue, I repeated the question back to my relative in hopes of buying myself some time to come up with a better reply. "What? When are we going to have a baby?" I squeaked out.

A male friend of Mark's once explained to me that when a man answers a question with "What?" it's like oxygen to them, giving their brains a chance to figure out how to answer the question or get out of the situation altogether. It wasn't until we were in the baby-creating mode that I fully understood and implemented the "What?" response.

That simple "What?" gave me extra seconds to navigate through difficult questions and observations: "When are you going to have a baby?" "Don't you want children?" "Boy, it takes you a long time to get pregnant!" And so on and so on. Of course, the "What?" tactic would only take me so far. Though good for use against surprise attacks, it earned only mere seconds. Then it would be back to me standing there, mouth half-open, panicked, searching the room for Mark to come and rescue me. At that stage, I was paralyzed by both the question and the anticipation of being questioned. This fear kept me home many nights.

Then Mark had a brilliant idea. Enter lucky Strategy Thirteen: The "Elevator Speech."™*

Mark uses this communication technique in one of our seminars. Through this seminar, Mark helps salespeople and financial advisors create a compelling thirty-second script to explain what they do and why a potential client might want to learn more about their services. The goal is to create a quick speech that will get your point across to someone in the time it takes for an elevator to go from one floor to the next.

Mark's brilliant idea was to apply this strategy to answering the questions about our plans for creating a family. This method worked wonders for me and took away the feelings of dread I'd attached to attending group functions. Being armed with a script will give you a feeling of security, and will empower you enough to avoid those emotional breakdowns that can leave you in tears and gasping for breath.

Putting It into Practice

The "Elevator Speech" also incorporates the strategy of visualization (see Strategy Three on page 21). You'll be rehearsing for such

* *Adapted from "The Elevator Speech" from* The Product Is You *by Mark Magnacca, pp 45-61.*

exchanges and preparing yourself to be confident at future family gatherings and other social events.

- On a sheet of paper, write out the question you hear most often or the one you dread the most. For example (a common favorite!) "So, when are you going to have a baby?"

- Take your time and think about some rational responses to that question that will put an end to the conversation, with no hard feelings on either end. Here are a few examples that we used and some that were shared by the couples who have attended our seminars:

  - "Babies come when babies come"
  - "I would love to have a baby; sometimes it isn't as easy as it seems."
  - "We have a whole team of people working on it."
  - "It's a long story."
  - "Not right now, but you'll be the first person I call when we do."

- Try to come up with a few of your own. Keep in mind the various people or family members who might be asking the question, and be prepared for follow-up questions. Remember that your answer should be gentle but firm.

- Now close your eyes and visualize yourself using the responses that you came up with. Notice which response feels or sounds the best to you during your mental movie.

- Then repeat your answer again and again until you feel comfortable saying it. Try practicing your "Elevator Speech" in front of the mirror. You could even practice this with your partner. Perhaps you might want to take turns asking the question and each of you responding with your individual "Elevator Speeches."

Another job well done! Now you're ready for any baby-related interrogation!

fourteen

Ducking and Dodging

I was sitting in our living room waiting for Mark to get home. It had been a trying day, and I was longing to share—actually, vent about—the day's events. The rumble of the garage door opening sent me out of my seat like a shot. I was at the door in seconds, swinging it open, my thoughts swirling in my head.

"Hey, baby, it's great to see you," Mark said, hugging me.

"Hey, baby! I've been waiting for you all day," I said with urgency. Then the floodgates opened.

"Mark, when they came to put the new floor in today, they didn't move the furniture or hang sheets in the door opening. I thought part of the fee for the flooring included them moving the furniture out! You know, if the sales guy had told us that there was going to be such a mess, I would have prepared the room better. I moved all the stuff I could by myself, but I would have covered and prepared the room differently. I'm thankful that we're getting the floor redone, but my goodness, what a mess! Look, there's a thin coat of dust all over the house, and I've cleaned it once already. I even had to take down the curtains and wash them. All this about the floor, and then there was work stuff that I can't even begin to tell you about, and—most upsetting of all—I got my period today, which just sent me over the edge. Look at the house; it's a mess!"

Stopping to take a breath, I looked at Mark. His eyes had glossed over, and I knew I had lost him back at "I thought part of the fee for the flooring..." He swung into "Mr. Fix-It" mode. "Give me the phone. I'll call the guy right now and talk to him about this. He certainly didn't meet my expectations."

Before he could find the phone, I was at it again. "Look at the countertop; I'm never going to get all this dust out of here. It's sawdust from the subfloor. They used a circular saw to cut the floor out. Did you know that they were going to do that?"

"No, Kristen, that's not what Mike, the floor guy, explained to me. Where's the phone?" Mark asked patiently.

Feeling better because I had gotten some of my frustration out, I looked at the kitchen and realized I could give it another wipe-down and it would be fine, that office work could be tackled tomorrow, and that my period coming was the cause of most of my negativity. It had all seemed so overwhelming until I was able to talk about it, and I felt so much better after my verbal purging. I took a deep breath.

On the other hand, Mark's annoyance was reaching the high end of the scale. "Wait till I get that guy on the phone," he sputtered out, still searching for the phone.

"No, don't call him. It's okay," I said as I reached for his hand.

"What do you mean, it's okay?" Mark said, by now utterly confused. "Kristen, you just said that they didn't do a good job and the house is a mess. I need to talk to him!"

"Yes, you do—but not now. It's okay. I'm so upset about today, especially my period coming, and the fact that we're going to have to talk about our next step again," I said, taking a deep breath and feeling almost refreshed enough to take on all the day's speed bumps.

Mark looked at me like I had two heads, and reached for his PalmPilot to get the floor store's phone number.

"It's okay, Mark, really—you don't need to call now. Let me clean off the table and we'll eat," I said, regaining my composure.

My husband was so confused and now frustrated because he felt as though he needed to fix the floor situation, address the work issues, talk about me getting my period, and come up with another way for us to get pregnant all at the same time.

In effect, I had just taken the monkey off my back and put it on Mark's. Now he felt burdened and overwhelmed, when all I had really wanted was for him to listen. I wanted Mark to hear out my frustrations, meet me emotionally, and acknowledge my feelings. In a sense, I wanted him to act like a woman, which was impossible. So instead of feeling like Mark understood me, I felt as though he thought I couldn't solve problems effectively. Meanwhile, he felt that he was failing me because he wasn't able to fix what he viewed as a problem.

After numerous conflicts like this, which stemmed from misunderstanding each other, we worked out a strategy to help us both feel supported, understood, and loved. It has had a very positive impact on our marriage. Now when I need to vent, I give Mark a heads-up that all he needs to do is listen to me. This made things easier for him because it allows him, for a brief moment, to focus on what I am saying instead of immediately creating a plan to fix my problems. It took some time before this became a habit, but when it did, the setup changed. Mark now asks me at the beginning of an exchange if all I need him to do is listen, and—once he knows the rules of engagement—he can deal with my verbal barrage.

Putting It into Practice

It's important to acknowledge from the start that there are different needs to be met when we share or update our partner on what is happening in our lives. So this strategy has three parts: one for the woman, one for the man, and one for both of them. For the most part, women want to be heard and understood. Men want to solve problems—their own, their friends', and their partner's. It is very difficult for men to just listen without taking action. They view their purpose in life to be providing for others and taking care of situations, and when they find their skills are not needed, it creates conflict between the parties.

For women
When you just want to vent, start out by giving specific directions to your male partner or listener:

"You don't have to fix any of this, I just want you to listen."

This is a clear indication to the man about the type of communication coming his way.

For men
This is probably best explained by using a boxing analogy. You are in the ring, facing your opponent (not that your partner is your opponent in real life, but for the purpose of this exercise, stick with me

for a minute), and you have your gloves on. The opponent throws the first shot, and you bend to the right to dodge the hit. The second shot is thrown, and you bend to the left and dodge that one, too. Just as if you're in the ring, you duck and dodge all the verbal shots your partner is throwing your way. You're light on your feet and you let them all go by, repeating to yourself, "I don't have to fix that one, I'm just going to listen and let it fly by me." As your partner vents, maintain eye contact with her and shake or nod your head appropriately. This will earn you enormous "great-husband" points while this exchange is happening. (This Duck-and-Dodge strategy is adapted from a similar concept proposed by Dr. John Gray, author of *Men Are from Mars, Women Are from Venus*.)

For women and men
Step Three involves acknowledgment from both sides. The woman says something like, "Thank you so much for listening. I know it's hard for you just to listen, and I feel so much better." Now the man expresses his appreciation for her ordeals of the day by saying something like: "Boy, that must have been difficult for you," "Do you need a hug?" and/or "C'mere, babe. Sorry you had such a lousy day."

Implementing this strategy takes time and practice, but once you both get the hang of it, you will notice the carry-over effect of better communication and a stronger connection.

Check the Weather

You can set your clock by my morning rituals. Up at 6:00 AM and into the bathroom to brush my teeth. At 6:10, I shuffle into my office, flip open my laptop, and hit my "Favorites" bar on my Web browser to check the weather.

"Rain again today! Ugh!"

Then, by 6:20, I'm off to my closet for the appropriate clothes.

"It's going to rain today along with high winds," I whisper. (One of my lesser-known roles in our marriage is Mark's personal weather girl.) I just hear a grunt in reply from the darkness of our room.

Mark and I could be a case study for the theory that opposites attract. I'm a morning person; he's a night owl. I'm happy to be alive in the morning and can accomplish a day's work before 10:00 AM. He's a slow starter and has a difficult time getting up and going.

"I hope your plane gets off okay. You might want to call ahead to see if there are any delays," I suggest. Another grunt from the darkness.

Mark thinks I'm obsessed with the weather and, in a way, I am. When you live in New England, you have to be prepared for anything:

snow, sleet, rain, high winds, and, on rare occasions, sunshine—all in one day!

In a sense, the same can be said for couples trying to have a baby. There's so much going on in each person's mental atmosphere that you never really know what mood, interpretation, or reaction to expect. By keeping the lines of communication open, you can better forecast the emotional weather of your relationship.

When Mark and I fail to communicate regularly, our relationship clearly suffers. During the months when we were focused on creating a baby, it didn't matter whether Mark was away on business or sitting right across from me at the dining room table: If we weren't making efforts to connect, we were only making things worse. Our company requires Mark to travel extensively. The separation is difficult and creates tension, but when we're communicating the distance seems manageable.

When we were trying to have a baby, we fell into a lack of regular communication that heightened our frustrations and formed a painful gap between us. I felt alone in the quest to create our family. Our lack of verbal connection left me only guessing what the situation meant to Mark, and I never even came close to his true perceptions.

That concept of projecting meaning upon the other person worked both ways. Mark would perceive my loneliness as anger toward him and feel compelled not only to try to fix it but also to protect himself. Not communicating created unnecessary stress for both of us.

"If you don't tell me what's going on, I start making things up in my head and they're worse than what they actually are," Mark commented one day. It became painfully obvious that we needed a strategy for maintaining a verbal connection, but we weren't sure how to go about it.

Not long after this discussion, on one of my morning trips into my office to check the weather, a light-bulb moment revealed to me a perfect solution: We could mimic my morning routine of checking the weather by checking each other's emotional weather! I decided to ask Mark to call me three times a day.

Mark received my request with a blank stare. His interpretation of my idea was that these three calls would consist of lengthy conversations during which I would go into every detail of what was happening with me at the current moment and he was supposed to fix it! Of course, that wasn't where I was going with this strategy, so I reminded him that he was armed with the concept of ducking and dodging and would only have to listen and understand.

Once Mark got used to the idea, it didn't take long for us to fall into a comfortable check-in rhythm. We began our "weather checks" with telephone calls. For us, voicemail messages worked because just listening to Mark's voice was a reminder that he was thinking of me and that we were a team! Mark would call me in the morning, at lunch, and then on the way home. It got to a point that it was habit for him to call; it became part of his daily routine.

As technology changed, so did we, and we eventually progressed to high-tech communications. Mark would e-mail me and I, in turn, would send a digital message back on his phone or respond by e-mail.

Now that we've implemented this strategy, we've learned that most of our miscommunications can be averted by *over*communicating—by having several quick check-ins throughout the day, using the same amount of time and effort that it takes to check the weather. These weather checks fulfill two needs: the woman's desire to share and talk about her day, and the man's desire to make his wife happy and feel as though he is a good husband. Sounds pretty basic, but fulfilling these needs creates a strong foundation for marriage.

The bonus effect of checking in is that the process of verbal connection, which is so necessary for women, gets broken down over the course of the day, becoming more manageable for the male to listen in parts rather than being bombarded with information all at once after work. This shortening also provides for a smoother time when the couple is physically together, which—in the typical case for the male partner—equals being "physically" together.

A therapist friend of mine said with a great big hearty laugh that it's God's great joke: Women need to feel connected before they have sex—by talking—and men feel connected by having sex. It's like the dog chasing its tail.

It took Mark a while to understand that for me, verbal connection is needed to form any intimate connection, and he meets my needs head-on so that I'll be open to connecting physically and meeting his needs.

Putting It into Practice

Chances are you both have busy and varying schedules, so it's a good idea to call a "marital meeting" to discuss the terms of your "weather check." For me, it was necessary to begin negotiations with Mark to connect three times during the day, really only needing one or two, because I knew he would want to barter me down.

During your meeting, discuss what time of day works the best for each party. Do you want to check in by phone three times a day? Or is a quick call at lunch enough? Who makes the first contact? Is a voicemail message sufficient? Other couples find that using only e-mail to stay connected works the best for them. Finding the appropriate method of communication will make this a pleasure. With all the new gadgets out there to let you "reach out and touch someone," the world is your oyster!

What you do when you make contact is up to you both. Emotional check-ins are so important, especially during baby-creating mode and high-tech intervention. Remember, you're checking in briefly during the day to see what your partner might need for support and to get a clear picture of what you might be needing for inclement emotional weather...your emotional umbrella or stormy galoshes.

You could possibly just need to lift the other person's spirits by sending the other person an e-mail joke or shifting attention to the latest office gossip. Use this time to get things off your chest if you need to. But be brief, though; you can discuss how to handle the outrageous electricity bill over dinner. Remember—you're just checking in.

If you are skeptical about this strategy, I encourage you to try it for a month, especially during the time that you are in the "waiting" period to see if all your efforts resulted in a positive conception.

It's simple—but powerful. Just like the weather.

Reflective Listening

*T*he store had been a neighborhood supermarket for fifty years. The local residents would walk to the store and, after they purchased their items, the delivery boy would bring their bags to their homes so that they would not have to struggle. There was great uncertainty, mostly among the older residents of the neighborhood, when I decided to renovate the structure and turn it into a preschool/learning center. After all, change is difficult at any age, and as a group they were very vocal about their concerns.

It was the summer of 1986, and I was twenty-two years old. I teetered on a ladder, stretching to paint the upper portion of a mural on the side of the long rectangular building. I was covered in the green paint I was using to depict a long blade of grass that would be the resting place for a cricket, which was the mascot for the preschool, Cricket's Corner Learning Center, Inc. Out of the corner of my eye, I noticed a man with a dog slowly walking directly toward me; you could almost see his words dancing in his head, sizing me up and appraising the situation.

I felt my body go into fight-or-flight mode, and my cheeks turned red from the external, and my internal, heat. The wall I was painting received direct sunlight, and the sunbeams were bouncing off the freshly painted bright-yellow building, intensifying the heat.

The man stopped at the base of my ladder, squinting up into the sun at me. "You know I shopped at this market all my life, and now you're coming here and what do you expect us to do?" He was venomous.

"Well, more people should have shopped here when the store was open and the owner would have been able to stay in business," I shot back. "It's not my fault they shut their doors." My response surprised even me, since I'm normally considerably more empathetic to others.

"How do you know how many of us shopped here? You aren't from here and you'll never fit in," was his final response. With that, he turned and left, his little dog's paws moving quickly to keep up with his exasperated pace.

That didn't go very well, I thought to myself. As the man stomped away, I felt like I had lost a perfect opportunity to introduce the school to a resident and become part of the neighborhood. I could see him more clearly with each step he was taking away from me. He was angered by the change and needed to tell me off because he viewed me as the source of the problem. Instead of seeing him as a grouchy old man, I should have recognized him as someone dealing with change and trying to communicate his feelings about it.

I asked myself how I could have handled the situation differently and realized that the same technique that I try to apply daily to preschoolers and other people in my life would have created a different outcome to my meeting with my neighbor. The technique is one I'd learned from my college psychology class and it is called "reflective listening."

The next day, when the man with the dog came walking by again, I stepped out to greet him, wanting to start over again with my new neighbor.

"I just wanted to come and properly introduce myself to you. My name is Kristen and I'm the owner of the preschool. I want to apologize to you about yesterday; I have to say that I did get hot under my collar. After thinking about what you said, it sounds to me that you're pretty upset about the market closing."

"I've been going to this market all my life! My wife and I would walk down every day and get the things we needed for dinner. We were close friends with the owners. First my wife passed, now they closed the market and they moved." He wasn't grouchy anymore, just sad and lonely.

"Boy, it sounds as though you've been through a lot in a short time. No wonder you were upset with me." My heart broke for him.

"Yeah, I guess so."

"How long how long were you married?"

"Forty-two years."

"Wow, do you have any good tips for staying married that long?" (I put the reflective listening aside for a moment to get the inside scoop!)

"Yes. Marry your best friend, because when things happen you always have someone."

"Do you feel as though you have no one now?"

He started to tear up. "Yes," he whispered.

"I know the feeling, I'm pretty young to be opening a business, and not too many people here are open to me changing the market into a preschool. It can be discouraging," I confided.

"I'll let them know that you're okay."

"I'll tell you what, I'll be here every day and I would appreciate it if you would wave to me when you walk by, that way at least I will know one person."

He shrugged his shoulders and turned to walk off. For years after that exchange, my new friend would stop by the front window and wave to me every morning. I felt as though I had someone looking out for the school, and I think it gave him a routine for the day.

Reflective listening is a way of helping someone explain themselves or their situation by empathizing with what they are saying while showing that you understand their feelings. It's like holding a verbal mirror up to the person so that they can hear back what they said, which will hopefully provide them with the ability to solve their own problem or concern. It also reassures them that you heard what they said and that you acknowledge what is important to them. Using reflective listening has payoffs for both parties. In the case of my irate neighbor, once I acknowledged and understood his resistance to change, our relationship changed and we became friendly. I got support from a community member, and he got recognition of his status in the neighborhood.

Putting It into Practice

Reflective listening is a powerful tool in a marriage. In reflective listening, you act as a mirror for your partner, reflecting back to him his feelings, emotions, or concerns. It's a form of give-and-take that encourages your partner to open up to you, thereby keeping your lines of communication open. All you have to do is remember the five R's:

Recognize: In the heat of a conversation in which a person is sharing something that is upsetting or hurtful to them, stop for a moment, recognize the opportunity, and instruct yourself to begin the reflective listening process.

Remind: Remind yourself that you are going to listen to the person's quandary and speak back their feelings to them. Make eye contact.

Reflect: Being the mirror, isolate the most important feelings being expressed, or the core of the problem, and start your short response back by beginning your statement with, "It sounds like you're saying you feel that . . ." or "Are you saying . . . ?"

Retreat: Step back and give the person time to acknowledge what you said and come to a solution on his or her own. By giving space and time, you are giving permission for the person to think or just feel what they are feeling.

Request: The notion of requesting I learned from Mark. He would do all of the above and then ask this wonderful question: "Are you asking me to help now?" The process would meet both our needs. I was allowed to talk about the situation and feel as though I was heard. On the occasions that the process of talking through the situation didn't result in a solution, Mark would have my permission to assist in solving the problem because he asked first if he was invited in to help.

This process may be awkward for the both of you at first, but with practice, it will flow easily. Just remember: Be the mirror.

seventeen

The Honey-Do List

*T*he **rolling motion of the boat** was not as debilitating as I thought it would be. We had been on this cruise for two days, and I felt as though I finally had my sea legs under me. Among the list of activities we had chosen for the day was skeet shooting off the back of the ocean liner.

Scanning the people standing in line, I noticed I was the only woman waiting for a turn at shooting the clay disk. The sailor in charge of loading the rifle and releasing the clay pigeons got a little annoyed when it was my turn.

"Have you ever shot a rifle before?"

"Nope," I replied.

His attitude was not what was advertised in the cruise brochure. He roughly positioned the rifle onto my shoulder and placed my fingers in the appropriate spots.

The weight of the rifle was more than I anticipated; my left hand drifted downward from the full weight of the barrel. I called out,

"Pull!" and, forcing the rifle upward, I followed the clay disk with the nose of the barrel and shot the gun. I missed the target and was propelled backwards from the recoil. The impact of the butt of the rifle on my shoulder smarted more than I'd thought it would, but I motioned to the sailor to release another disk. By the end of my third try at shooting, I had gotten the hang of it—the stance, the balance of the gun, and the bracing for the recoil.

That night, back in our cabin, I noticed Mark leaning over the daily activity sheet that had been placed in our room the night before.

"The midnight buffet—check; daily run—check; skeet shooting—check;" he said as he crossed off the words on the list.

"My shoulder can attest to that!" It bore the brunt of my stubbornness and was turning an interesting shade of black and blue.

"Conga line—check; daily excursion—check. All done." Mark reached for a folder bearing the cruise line's emblem and carefully slipped the sheet inside it. As I watched him, I noticed two other sheets in there, already checked and placed there for safekeeping.

Closing the covers, Mark glanced my way. "All done?" I asked.

"Hey, I think I'm doing good being disconnected from work. I just need to feel that sense of accomplishment."

For some reason, Mark's habit of checking off his daily activities stuck with me. We used this strategy on weekends to motivate him to focus on what needed to be done around the house. Together, we would write a list and take a break after each task to check it off. It goes back to the fact that Mark moves toward pleasure, and he got pleasure from watching his list dwindle down to nothing. He needed to see what was done and what needed to be completed.

Three years into our attempts at creating our family, our marriage was just as bruised as my shoulder had been from the rifle—from the time it took to uncover the physical issues impeding our attempts to get pregnant, our failed two intrauterine insemination attempts, and then the joy of hearing that we were successful crushed when I was rushed to the hospital for emergency surgery that resulted in the loss of our baby and damage to one of my fallopian tubes. But in the case of our marriage, the cause of the bruising was invisible. It was the pure emotional trauma that we both attacked so differently while trying in vain to help the other person. We had sought out professionals to help us navigate the unknown territory of infertility, we asked for guidance from our doctors, we went to marriage counseling, and still we were drifting apart like the dividing wake behind our beloved cruise ship.

Logically, I knew that every marriage had its own flow and cycle, and when the flow of energy is compromised by stressors—such as getting a new house or a new job, attempting to have a child, or dealing with a miscarriage—these life events change how you communicate and view yourself, your partner, and your marriage.

We both realized that we were in conflict, and we were trying in vain to fix the problem. To make matters worse, in the midst of it all we weren't communicating, we weren't participating in each other's day. We lived in the same house and mourned our circumstances separately.

One morning, I woke up and realized that the pregnancy we had lost might not be the only tragedy that we could encounter, that our marriage was teetering dangerously close to falling overboard without a life preserver. I knew I had to do something. I wanted to get back to the point where we both felt good about our partnership. Remembering how we used to talk about everything and anything, and how that made everything feel so real, I desperately wanted that feeling back. Then I asked myself, what did Mark do that made me feel loved, appreciated, and secure?

The answer came back to me in images. Our first date popped into my mind: We had talked the night away. The images fast-forwarded through our numerous dinners, which included talking, talking, and more talking. Next, I thought back to our old nightly routine of going to bed together, reading and sharing with each other the words on the pages in our hands. These images and memories freshly in mind, I pulled out a stack of colored 3x5 cards from my office, and picked a bright pink card off the top. On the top line in the left-hand corner, I started to number the lines. Then I wrote down the three things I needed from Mark that day. I was hopeful that they would bring back the lost feeling of connection we'd had:

* Call me three times today
* Have dinner with me
* Go to bed with me and read

There it was. That was what I needed, three things from Mark, and they all boiled down to being together: physically together, sharing again, the normal relationship things. On the back of the card I wrote a line from our wedding vows: "Through sickness and health, in good times and bad. June 10, 1995."

The next step was to sell this to Mark. I greeted him with coffee and the bright pink card. At first, as usual, he gave me a blank stare as I explained how I thought this would work. Each morning, we could exchange cards with three things we needed from each other that day, and at the end of the day, we could hand back the checked-off card. And, if we felt like it, we could write a quote on the back. It was something we both could do that would give us a sense of fixing what wasn't working.

Mark still looked a little dazed, but then it was his turn to write down what he needed. On his first card he wrote the following:

* A proper greeting when I get home
* Remind me why you married me
* Ask me about my day and listen with interest

It was all so doable! I knew the proper greeting was important for Mark, and I withheld it because I knew it bothered him! Remembering why I married him was easy, and to listen was what I longed for, too, but my bitterness had taken away any generosity of spirit I might have had to be the first person to break the ice.

It was amazing how this piece of paper changed our energy toward our marriage. Instead of indifference, we had connection. It got to the point that we were surprising each other with cards in unusual places—taped on the fridge, pinned to the shower, and in our giddiness we took our requests to the extreme.

One night, as he was driving up the hill to our house, Mark decided to fulfill his third call of the day to me and called me from his cell phone.

"I'm coming home to you, baby," he said. I could feel his mood shift from not wanting to come home, to anticipating us being together.

"Yippee!" I opened the door and ran to our driveway to wait for his car.

As he turned the corner into our driveway, I proceeded to jump up and down and scream, "You're home, you're home!" Now, *that* was a proper greeting! He was very embarrassed and, although he didn't admit it, flattered.

That night after dinner, while handing me back my lime-colored index card, Mark smiled and said, "I feel like a great husband."

"You know what, baby? You are!" And we locked each other in a tight hug.

I look back at how we struggled to find someone or something to help us communicate and cope with all that had happened to us on the journey to create a family, and it came down to communicating what we needed and not withholding what the other needed. We'd been playing "mind-reader," assuming that the other person should know what we wanted or needed without having to say it out loud. Then we'd become resentful when the other person wasn't fulfilling our needs. I felt that Mark already knew what I needed, but wasn't taking steps to help me. I certainly didn't know what Mark needed, and he wasn't telling me. The Honey-Do List strategy was a clear-cut way of getting our needs met and communicating them in a non-threatening manner.

We started using this strategy four years ago. We exchanged cards daily for three months, then, when we felt as though we had integrated each other's needs into our daily lives, we moved away from this strategy for a short period. When Mark's schedule required him to be away for days at a time, we would write out the appropriate number of cards and keep up the Honey-Do List even though we were miles apart. Continuing to use this strategy even when we were miles apart kept the momentum going and kept us connected during the separation.

Now we use our 3x5 cards as a fallback strategy to cut short marital misunderstandings or when one of us is feeling unappreciated, unloved, or misunderstood. I saved our cards in a filing box and sometimes pull out Mark's old cards and remind myself what it takes for me to meet his needs.

Putting It into Practice

Pick up a packet or two of 3x5 index cards. We think the brightly colored ones are fun, but of course that's up to you.

The basic rules are straightforward: Every morning, each partner dates a card and writes three things that he or she needs from the other person that day. On the back of the card you can write a quote or a saying that you feel is appropriate. Then exchange your cards. Have some fun with this: Try hiding the cards around the house, putting one on your partner's dashboard, slipping another into a briefcase (make sure it's easy to find).

During the day, as you fulfill your partner's needs, check them off the list.

At the end of the day, return the checked-off card to your partner. If for some reason a request hasn't been completed, then that person is responsible for explaining why and requesting another day to fulfill that obligation.

This strategy truly helped save our marriage. And other couples have found success with it, too. The day after Mark and I presented our Honey-Do List during a seminar, I received the following e-mail from a woman who was in the group. She wrote:

"With my 3x5 card in hand, I ventured off today feeling SO MUCH MORE connected to my husband than I have in months. Just by reading his first request, 'Wake me and say I love you BEFORE you go to work'...made me feel like he really DOES still care. Thank you and Mark for this, Kristen. We intend to keep this journey going with these cards, as we continue our infertility journey. It has been a long five years, and what you said last night really stuck. We both thank you most sincerely!"

Albert Einstein once said, "Everything should be made as simple as possible, but not one bit simpler." We should all take his lead and incorporate his philosophy into strengthening our relationships.

eighteen

Do You Want to Be Right, or Do You Want to Be Loving?

"Kristen, I have to tell you about this woman who broke the board last night." Mark had excitement in his voice. He was referring to part of one of the seminars we present, titled "Breakthrough." We use several metaphors to explain that by following the behavior and patterns of someone who has obtained results similar to those you desire, you can accelerate your own path toward achieving your goals. It's like following the recipes of a great chef. As an exercise, we give participants an opportunity to break pine boards with their bare hands.

Mark continued after a gulp of coffee. "She was this little person, and when she got up to the front of the room she was visibly shaking. I leaned over to her and said, 'You know, I wouldn't have picked you do to this if I didn't know you could.'"

Well, you could have pushed me over with a feather. These compassionate and caring words came out of the same man who, during a conversation prior to leaving for that same seminar, was hell-bent on determining which one of us was *wrong*. Or, really, was bent on proving that *I* was wrong! The notion of being loving and showing compassion and understanding for my feelings apparently never crossed his mind. But, surprisingly enough, only a few hours later he was able to see right through this woman and comfort and console her lovingly to the point where she took positive action.

My mouth hung open. "That's amazing," was all I could say.

Mark thought I was referring to the transformation of the woman in the story.

So I continued, "You do have the ability to know what to say and to be compassionate and understanding! It's amazing to me that you can do this for a strange woman and not for your wife."

It was apparent that I was still feeling bitter and hurt; Mark's sharing just sent me over the edge. I now found myself bracing for round two of our argument from the night before, pushing the full weight of my body into the floor. I could almost hear the wood beneath my feet bend from the pressure. Mark stood on the other side of the kitchen island. It was as if our kitchen had turned into a tennis court, but, instead of tennis balls, we began volleying hostilities across the surface.

"That's because she listened and wasn't trying to make me wrong," Mark shot back.

"I wasn't trying to make you wrong; you were insinuating that I was wrong," I said, lobbing the unproductive volley back at Mark.

"I was not!" Mark shot back again.

We were like two five-year-olds protecting ourselves.

"Oh yeah, you're fat and ugly and your mom dresses you funny, too," was all I could come up with next. To tell you the truth, I was beginning to forget what initially started the argument and was focusing solely on my feelings. The outcome didn't really matter; I wasn't going to let my tennis opponent win! I was convinced he was wrong and I was right, and he was convinced I was wrong and he was right.

Isn't it amazing how two rational people can treat the person they love most in the world with such harshness, not to mention stupidity?

We both started to laugh.

"What were we arguing about in the first place, anyway?" I asked, deciding to let go of my desire to win.

"I don't really remember. Oh yeah, we were talking about why the bathroom is cold and why we didn't put the new thermostats in the bathroom. You thought it was because I didn't want to add to the expense, and I thought it was because they couldn't go in the bathroom because of moisture."

"And because I was responsible for getting this project done, I felt attacked because you were complaining about how cold it was during your morning shower, when all along it was you who didn't want to spend the money on the new thermostats for the bathrooms and you blamed it on me," I retaliated.

I had slipped far away from being loving, shocking myself back to reality.

"Let's start over," I sighed. "The problem is the cold bathroom. I wish it was handled differently from the beginning but it wasn't, so I'll call the electrician again and ask him to come back to see if the thermostats can be replaced. If they can't, I'll ask about alternatives that can get us to our desired outcome—a warm bathroom. I'll run the cost by you prior to the final okay." Although I hadn't proven who actually was wrong, I felt good about the solution.

"Thanks," he replied.

"And by the way, you did a nice job handling the woman breaking the board. You should be proud of yourself, even though sometimes you still do dress funny."

The vying to be right was an issue that kept creeping into our marriage, and it reared its ugly head much more when we were attempting to create our family. Then one day when I was having my astrological chart done, I brought this issue up. I was wondering if it was it because of some planetary alignment. Were our signs just incompatible for this issue? It turned out that the planets had nothing to do with our desire to blame each other when things didn't go smoothly. The woman doing my astrological reading told me that the matter of "being right" is a big issue for many couples. She then shared a quote: "Do you want to be right or loving?" I knew the quote and had tried to live its message, but, for some reason, both Mark and I found it hard to implement it in a heated discussion.

I asked myself what was behind the blaming: Fear of inadequacy? Fear of not being protected? I couldn't understand my feelings behind the silly thermostat argument, so I tried to peel off one more layer of the onion.

Just like the woman who feared being chosen to participate in the seminar, I feared that if I was wrong, I was inadequate. For me, that meant I was not self-sufficient, and if I couldn't handle everything, I would not be in control. In this light, the blaming was about trying to gain control. Hmm, very interesting. So I'd figured it out. Now what? I had uncovered the *why* for my behavior and needed the *how*. How not to try to make Mark wrong?

It's uncanny the way the universe sends you insights just when you need them. I was engaged in a conversation with a friend who is a family therapist with an amazing talent for helping people peel back the layers to see what motivates specific behaviors. We were discussing the blame game in marriages and my friend hit the nail on the head with a profound saying. "You buy your innocence with other people's guilt," he told me. In relationships, we sometimes try to meet our own unconscious needs—to feel in control, in my case—by proving we're in control, and that our partner is not. It reminded me of a quote from the Book of Matthew in the Bible: "And why beholdest thou the mote that is in thy brother's eye, but considerest not the beam that is in thine own eye?" It's so much easier to see the faults of others than it is to look at how we contributed to a negative situation. We resort to blaming to prove our innocence.

Putting It into Practice

How can you consistently choose to be loving? The R's to the rescue again:

Recognize: During a heated conversation, recognize that somewhere in the problem-solving process you've started playing the blame game. You might feel like you're being attacked, hear an accusing tone from your partner, or notice you and your partner physically bracing yourselves.

Remind: Remind yourself that both you and your partner are doing the best you can, and then say out loud, "I'm doing the best I can, and I think you are, too."

Request: Request a time-out.

Reflect: Ask yourself, what is the desired outcome? It could be to pay the bills and meet all the financial responsibilities or it could be to pick up the dry cleaning, or decide on the next step to create a child. Reflect on how this desired outcome can be reached without finger-pointing.

Reorganize: Loving, as defined by Encarta World English Dictionary, is an adjective meaning something is "done with enjoyment and careful attention." I love the sound of "careful attention." Look through loving eyes and reorganize the steps necessary to meet the desired outcome.

Tennis is always so much more enjoyable on a sunny day, and so is a marriage with a foundation of love.

Red-Flag Phrases

*I*t was one of those obligatory events that Mark was expected to attend, and he was trying to persuade me to go with him.

"It will be just a quick cocktail followed by dinner." Mark tried to make his voice encouraging.

"I've been to your 'quick cocktails followed by dinner,' and they last for months," I replied.

"No, really, Kristen—it would be good for you to meet him and his staff. I'll be working closely with him for the next few months, and I want to get your read of the situation."

"Can't I get a read on him over the phone?" I joked.

It had been such a long, hectic day and the added gloominess of the bleak winter weather made 4:30 in the afternoon feel like midnight. The last thing I wanted to do was leave our warm, holiday-bedecked house to face a wind-chill factor of two below zero and a cocktails-and-dinner party full of people I didn't know.

"Come on, Kristen, it'll be fun." Mark always says things will be fun because he thinks that will motivate me.

"I really don't want to go, Mark. Besides, I'll be the only female in a group of type-A men all vying for their turn in the spotlight!"

Then Mark pulled out the big guns. "It's really important to me."

I didn't need to reply. I just nodded and headed for my closet to find something appropriate for a business dinner.

Half an hour later, we were sitting in the bar waiting for our table. I wasn't going to ask why my presence at this restaurant was so important to him, but I knew it must have meant a lot since he was willing to pull out our "red-flag" phrase: "It's really important to me."

Those five words are like the "Get Out Of Jail Free" card in Monopoly. You use it sparely, strategically, and only for a very significant event. When Mark pulled out the red flag for this dinner, I knew that I hadn't understood the extent of his feelings about working with this new group. With those words, he was able to cut to the chase and make me realize I had to take action to meet his needs.

We started to use a red-flag phrase when we had difficulty communicating our true feelings about an upcoming event or a current situation in our lives (e.g., making a baby). Pulling the red-flag card works when it is truly imperative that the other person fulfills your desired request, or to drive home the magnitude of the point you are trying to make. In short, it is a stop sign that gets your partner to respect what you are saying.

"It's really important to me," is not the only red-flag phrase we use. "These pretzels are making me thirsty," carries an equal amount of weight in our marriage. The pretzel flag was born at a family event at my mother's house. Our lack of children had become a hot topic of discussion among our elderly relatives.

Lucky for us, we had practiced our "Elevator Speech" and it quickly rolled off Mark's tongue, but I was growing edgy and depressed after listening to probing questions all afternoon.

"I just want to leave, Mark," I said, looking at him longingly. "Can't we just leave?"

But Mark was looking over my shoulder as he was comforting me. He spotted our brother-in-law, who was heading to the park for a pick-up basketball game.

"You'll be fine," Mark said, and off he went to play basketball.

After we got home that night, I was wondering how I could have explained to Mark that even though we handled the situation well, emotionally I was not up to answering the same questions (again) about why we weren't pregnant yet. I knew Mark misunderstood how important it was for me to retreat to the safety of our home when I wanted to earlier in the day.

Later that night, as we snuggled on the couch and watched a rerun of *Seinfeld*, we couldn't stop laughing whenever one of the group said, "These pretzels are making me thirsty." It was a true "Aha!" moment for me. Although the phrase wasn't used in the same context as a signal to the other person, it just stuck with Mark and me.

"You know, Mark, I think we had a miscommunication before at my mom's. I really didn't want to stay anymore. I know that the questions about our childlessness came from a group of people who don't know what we go through each and every day to have a baby, but today, I wasn't equipped to handle it emotionally." I tried not to be upset with Mark and blame him for wanting to play basketball while I was in pain over our situation, but I really wanted him to know how I felt.

I continued. "How about the next time we're at a function and the other person wants to go, even if there is a lack of understanding about how much or why one of us wants to go, we say, 'Boy, these pretzels are making me thirsty.' That way we will both know that the other is at the breaking point."

"That's perfect, baby, and I'm so sorry," Mark replied. "I thought we handled the situation well and moved on from the comment. I didn't realize that it affected you so much—and, boy, are these pretzels making me thirsty."

It was a done deal. The Magnaccas had a new red flag, with a sprinkle of salt.

Putting It into Practice

Many couples already have some form of intimate language of their own. We know a couple who call each other "goob." We think they call each other that because chocolate and peanuts go so well together, but we'll never really know. That's what we're looking for here—some key word or phrase that reminds you of your intimacy with your partner, defines a situation or feeling, and immediately makes you both respond to the other's wishes with great respect.

Get together with your partner and jot down a few sayings that are already part of your family's private language. After creating a short list, mutually decide on which phrase seems to work best for you and integrate it into your decision-making or negotiating process. Each of you might want to pick your own individual "red-flag" phrase, or you might need several for various situations.

Once you both agree to the phrases, you must also agree to abide by the urgency they represent. Make a pact or a pledge to each other that when one person uses that phrase, the other must respect the request. And no crying wolf, either. This is a sacred bond between the two of you. It's like playing cards; you hold your hand close to your chest and play your most important cards only when you know they will have the greatest impact.

Using red-flag phrases has had profound effects on our understanding of each other and our communication. By listening and unconditionally complying to a request, we meet each other's needs and create what each of us desires most: a charmed marriage.

III

Rolling with the Changes

Keep Time in Perspective

$\mathcal{M}$y girlfriend sent me one of those annoying e-mails that, forward by forward, gets passed around the world. The subject line, "Why Women's To-Do Lists Never End," was the only reason I opened the e-mail.

According to the story, even with a focused to-do list, a woman is left at the end of the day feeling as though she didn't get enough done. During the process of completing her required tasks, she inadvertently gets sidetracked by life.

The e-mail went something like this (I'm inserting my real life here):

She starts off down the stairs to put a glass in the dishwasher before leaving for work. When she arrives in the kitchen, she notices the table wasn't wiped. She wipes the table and brings the dishtowel to the laundry area where she puts the towel in the washing machine, which completes a full load, so she presses the start button. Heading back to the dishwasher, she notices her husband's nightly snack dishes left by his favorite chair. Picking them up to add to the dish-washing load, she stops and folds the blanket that should be on the back of the chair. Finally putting the glass and snack dishes in the dishwasher, she notices that the rinse agent light is glowing on the washing machine and stops to add that in.

Grabbing her coat to go to work, she sees that the trash hasn't been taken out and begins to sort the recyclable paper, plastic, glass, and tin into their appropriate bins. She carries the trash outside, gets into her car, takes a deep breath, and wonders why she's feeling behind already. Glancing down, she sees that the low-fuel light is on and, sigh, she's off to the gas station! While reaching for her credit card en route to the gas station, she notices that the purple dry cleaning bag on the passenger seat, placed there by her spouse, is now her morn-ing companion for the ride to work. After wiping her hands off so as not to smell like gas, she decides to take the long way to her appointment so she can go through the drive-thru at the dry cleaners and ensure that the clothes will be ready in time for an upcoming business trip.

She arrives at the restaurant for her breakfast meeting just in time, requests to be seated, and waits a few seconds for her party to arrive. During those few moments she opens her day-runner and reviews her daily to-do list. Number One stares back at her: Stop at the post office to mail work packets. Oh, man, she thinks, I'll swing there afterward. The meeting goes well; she assembles her meeting action items and feels confi-dent that this relationship is a match. Jumping in her car, she drives to the post office, mails the packages, and purchases stamps for an upcoming mailing.

She arrives at her desk in time for a conference call, which goes well, and then turns her attention to an urgent situation that has developed regarding an upcoming speaking event. Her computer clock shows that it's after lunch; she'll eat later. She regroups to push ahead on her list of things to do. It's 2:30 in the afternoon, and only two things are crossed off. Feeling a bit of tightness in her chest, she fills her glass of water and starts making her calls, completing only two of the four after being interrupted a few times to answer inbound calls. She reminds herself she has a meeting with the graphic designer at 4:00 PM and realizes if she leaves now, she'll be able to make it to the bank to make a deposit on the way. Taking a few minutes to organize herself for the 4:00 meeting, she grabs the appropriate folders and some UPS packages that need to be put into the box before 5:00 PM for next-day delivery. With her coat on one arm, she reaches for her to-do list and dates the next sheet in the pad for tomorrow, transcribing numbers four to six on tomorrow's list. Now she feels a bit inadequate. How could she only have finished three things today?

Running out the door while putting her coat on, she's back in the car and arrives at the UPS box, double-checks that the envelopes are securely in the box, jumps back in the car, and arrives on time for her meeting. She signs off on the design of the brochure, okays the price for printing, and is off to the grocery store for dinner supplies.

Feeling tired and somewhat confused about how she so mismanaged her time that she didn't finish her to-do list for the day, she prepares dinner, does another load of laundry, and tidies up the house. Dragging a bit now, she heads upstairs to wash her face and put her pajamas on, but first she turns on the dishwasher, empties the laundry basket, refreshes the towels in the bathroom, reads her e-mails and responds to a few of them. At last she washes her face and climbs in bed, exhausted. She reaches for her journal and wonders how to start today's entry.

"I didn't really get that much done today. . ." she writes.

How far from the truth is *that*!?

Yet how true it is for all of us, especially women. We are in constant motion—doing, doing, doing—and accomplishing so much each and every day that enhances our lives, yet we feel as though we haven't done enough. How accurate the subject line was of that e-mail; we are never truly done with our doing. And this applies to men as well as women. Time keeps on running, running, running, and it seems it's always running away from us and we never seem to catch up.

But what we must keep in mind, the really important part, is that in our doing we are also being. By being, I mean being who we are as people, being part of the process of creating—and that includes creating a family and also being aware of both.

Putting It into Practice

How can you keep time in perspective? I believe that things happen for a reason and each of us is where we should be, doing exactly what we are supposed to be doing, at every moment in time. You can take the following measures and give yourself permission to be happy with the work you do.

Recognize: Tell yourself that you are in the *process* of creating your child, and you are right where you need to be today, doing exactly what you are supposed to be doing, and what you accomplish is enough. You've done enough.

Reassess: Just like when you are at work and, in the heat of doing what you are doing, you don't always notice your efforts, the same is true regarding the steps you are taking to make parenthood a reality. You might not think that you have done anything to move the ball closer to creating a family, but in reality you are! Have you eaten correctly? Yes! Taken your folic acid or vitamins? Yes! Your partner has on his boxers, correct? You're monitoring your cycle, and documenting the time of your ovulation, right? Of course you are! You've had blood tests and an ultrasound to assess your fertility cycle, right? All these are part of the process of creating and the concept of being in the moment. Appreciate yourself and your accomplishments.

Remind: Finally, remind yourself that what is consistent in any process is the beginning, middle, and the end, and as with all things, this process will come to an end. You're doing everything you can, starting at the beginning, working through the middle, and anticipating a positive ending.

twenty-one

Bring in the Consultants!

*A*t the urging of my friend Sarah, I made an appointment to see a craniosacral therapist. My tight jaw had been acting up, flaring into full-blown TMJ (Temporomandibular Joint) pain, and Sarah thought that the soft-touch physical therapy treatment would be just the right thing to correct the condition.

I had been experimenting with various alternative therapies to help not only with my jaw pain, but also with my infertility issues. I'd found an acupuncturist whom I'd been using and hadn't decided if it was right for me, but I was also doing meditation and focused relaxation and having good results. I swear, I felt like the poster girl for holistic approaches to whatever ails you.

Sarah was convinced that craniosacral therapy could also help with my infertility issues; the skillful therapist she recommended might be able to "clear the way" for a healthy pregnancy.

After receiving a warm welcome upon my arrival at the therapy center, I was escorted to a softly lit room, where soothing music was playing overhead. I climbed up on the table and lay on my back, feeling myself sink down deep into the thickly padded table. When Sarah's friend Lisa entered the room, she began the session by holding my ankles and feeling my body through her hands. At first it felt a little awkward, but as my body began to release into a deeper state of relaxation, I knew my ankles and the rest of my body were in the hands of a gifted healer. The relaxing treatment lasted a little under an hour.

When Lisa whispered into my ear that I should rest for a moment before leaving, I wished the treatment hadn't come to an end, but I followed instructions and allowed my body and senses to come back to a state of alertness. As soon as my feet hit the ground, I felt different. My body was in total alignment, feeling strange and wonderful all at once.

My body had never felt so centered before. I'd had massages that felt great, but this was a different level of alignment, as if Lisa had reforged the connection between my mind, body, and soul. I was hooked, and scheduled an appointment every two weeks.

That was years ago. Mark did not have as much faith in alternative therapies as I did. At his insistence, I was scheduled for a hysterosalpingogram around the same time. Mark thought it was important to determine if my fallopian tubes were functioning.

Over the course of my craniosacral treatments, I had gotten a sense that my tubes and reproductive organs were working through the emotional connection to the blockage, that there was a sense of leftover trauma from my earlier ectopic pregnancy. I knew I had a blockage throughout that region, but with each session I gained a greater sense of lightness there. For Mark, however, the correlation between the therapy and unblocking the tubes was hard to make.

I reluctantly went for the hysterosalpingogram, allowing them to shoot a harmless dye up through my cervix into my fallopian tubes via a catheter. A positive outcome for this test—the one I was expecting—would be if the dye went up through my uterus, out through each of my fallopian tubes, and spilled out into my abdominal cavity. Watching my test on the television screen in real time, however, proved that I was wrong; the dye did not spill out beyond my fallopian tubes. My stomach and reproductive organs were filled with a great sense of pain as, to no avail, the doctor injected more dye solution through the catheter to see if it could push loose the blockage that was impeding the way.

At my next visit with Lisa, I told her about the hysterosalpingogram and its disappointing result. "I don't feel any blockage, Kristen," Lisa replied with great certainty and directness.

"Then how do you explain the blockage of the dye?" I asked, feeling confused.

"Fear is a real thing, Kristen; the tube was in spasm, causing the dye to stop."

Even for me, that was hard to believe. I had seen it with my own two eyes: The dye had become trapped in my fallopian tubes and had not moved beyond them. I found it hard to believe that just my fear over the procedure would cause my tubes to go into such spasm that they would close! I would later come to realize just how much our emotional state can affect our physical function. Months later, I was in my reproductive endocrinologist's office reviewing the blood test that confirmed we were indeed pregnant. I queried him about the findings from the hysterosalpingogram. "The dye test showed that the tubes were blocked, so how do you explain our pregnancy?" I said.

Looking at both Mark and me, our reproductive endocrinologist first pointed up to the sky, insinuating that God played a huge role, then added that the test could have thrown the tube into spasm.

Spasm. Why didn't he say that was a possibility before? I sputtered out.

Throughout the journey to parenthood, Mark and I engaged the help of numerous consultants. They came in all forms and from all ranges of the therapeutic spectrum, including marriage consultants, acupuncturists, urologists, endocrine specialists, massage therapists, and personal coaches. We devoured books detailing Eastern and Western techniques, both holistic and traditional. With some consultants, we had individual sessions; with others we gained knowledge, such as how to incorporate relaxation-response techniques, and by attending seminars. I also called upon a friend who was a psychic, tried holographic repatterning, and visited a tarot card reader—just to name a few.

Mark and I had different approaches to deciding which consultants were the best for us. Mark viewed our situation more in black and white. I, on the other hand, became almost obsessive in my search for just the right alternative technique that would at last help us get pregnant, and I would try them all at least twice. This was partly due to my obsessive personality, but it also helped me cope with my feelings of powerlessness regarding our reproductive life. The act of "doing something" made me feel as though I was helping the cause or fixing the problem. I was crazed, trying to do *all* the alternative therapies, but finally felt the greatest benefits when I was doing just *one*—craniosacral therapy was the best for me.

Although not as convinced as I, Mark was a believer in the mind-body connection and alternative and complementary therapies, and

I was thankful he was able to acknowledge my need to work through the holistic buffet and achieve some semblance of balance in my treatments.

Listed at the end of this strategy are just a few of the consultants and therapy techniques Mark and I called on in our mission to become parents. You might find some of them helpful in your attempts at creating a family. Before you read over the list, take a moment to read the tips and recommendations below to help you choose your options.

Putting It into Practice

I encourage you to consider any *safe* alternative treatment that resonates with you. Here are some tips for evaluating these options before beginning treatment:

1. Notice how your body feels while you read the descriptions below. Questions sometimes answer themselves in the asking. Let one of the suggestions speak to you and invite you to try it. It might be a feeling or a vision, or maybe when you hear the description in your head it will call to you. (This is really accessing your intuition, which I'll discuss in Strategy Twenty-seven.) Listen for a clue to see which one is a match for you.

2. Communicate your feelings to your partner about the array of complementary choices. Friends of ours were open to some of the "stuff," but not to others. They would not go to see a marriage counselor, for example, because they associated going to marriage counseling with being in a dire situation, but they did go to a nurse counselor for guidance. It's all about what you and your partner

associate with the given terms; you might want to bring back the association game to help move the process along.

3. Keep in mind that there's so much more to these treatments than relaxation. It takes time, energy, and effort to work these alternative techniques. And be prepared to receive some off-handed comment about how all you have to do is relax and you'll get pregnant. (Have your "Elevator Speech" ready to reply to that one.) The meditation, craniosacral therapy, journaling, and everything else do elicit a relaxation state, but it's not just about sitting around with a piña colada while being fanned by a servant. It takes mental energy to apply Eastern healing practices and, most importantly, those brought up in a Western culture must first accept that there may be more to healing than simply taking drugs or enduring surgeries. You must appreciate the connection between your mind and your body if any of these approaches are to work.

4. A girl has a right to change her mind. (Boys do too!) If you set out on a course with one approach and find it's not the right one for you, don't feel as though it was unsuccessful. Chalk it up to experience and pick another or none at all. It's your decision to go holistic or not.

Acupuncture

Acupuncture is an ancient healing art developed over five thousand years ago in China and is recognized by the World Health Organization for effectively treating a variety of ailments. It is based on the theory that all disease is the result of imbalance in the body's energy, which can result in either physical or emotional illness. "Energy" includes both the blood and an invisible force called "Qi" (pronounced "chee"). Qi flows though the body in a system of pathways called "meridians," which correspond to the vital internal organs of the body. If there is a problem with a particular organ, symptoms may occur anywhere along its related meridian. These points are located where the Qi is concentrated. Acupuncture treatments adjust the flow of Qi and stimulate your body's own healing capabilities.

Acupuncture can be used for gynecology and infertility, for both men and women, for poor egg quality or implantation, miscarriages, PMS, irregular or painful periods, endometriosis, premature menopause, menopausal symptoms, low sperm count, and low sperm movement.

Craniosacral Therapy

Craniosacral Therapy (CST) is a gentle, hands-on method of evaluating and enhancing the functioning of a physiological body system called the craniosacral system—the membranes and cerebrospinal fluid that surround and protect the brain and spinal cord.

Using a soft touch, generally no greater than five grams, or about the weight of a nickel, practitioners release restrictions in the craniosacral system to improve the functioning of the central nervous system.

By complementing the body's natural healing processes, CST is used increasingly as a preventive health measure for its ability to bolster resistance to disease, and is effective for a wide range of medical problems associated with pain and dysfunction.

Massage Therapy

A great massage can make you feel as though you can touch heaven. It's a soft or deep pressure applied by hand to all of the body. The questions you have to ask yourself before going for your appointment are: Can you handle your body being touched by a stranger? And,

how much of your body do you want to expose? Some people leave
their underclothes on, others do not. It's up to you.

Meditation

Meditation is the act of quieting your body and mind while focusing
on one thing to create a sense of well-being. It can be done anywhere
and any time of the day that is convenient for you. There are different forms of meditation. The purpose of this practice is to create a
personalized system in which you focus on your oneness with the
universe and foster feelings of tranquility. Meditation takes patience
and practice, but the benefits are well worth the effort.

Personal Coach

A personal or professional coach works with clients to help them
understand their challenges or desires, develop goals, and create a
plan to achieve their desired results.

Reproductive Endocrinologist

A reproductive endocrinologist is a medical doctor who specializes in
infertility, working to help couples get pregnant. If you choose to see
one, make sure he or she is board-certified. How do you know if you
need to see one? The rule of thumb is that couples who have had
unprotected sex for more than a year without conceiving are considered infertile, and would do well to visit a reproductive endocrinologist. There are also special situations when you might consider
scheduling an appointment earlier than the one-year cut off. If you
have been exposed to DES (diethylstilbestrol) like I was, you may
want to get checked out early on. DES was given to women of my

mother's generation when they were threatening to miscarry. It causes numerous birth defects and affects baby girls' reproductive organs.

Urologist

A urologist is a physician who specializes in male and female urinary systems and the male reproductive organs. When we started investigating what was impeding our attempts at getting pregnant, we were told that the male factor is the easiest to rule out because it requires a noninvasive sperm analysis. The test showed a lower than normal result, and Mark was referred to a urologist, who was able to quickly identify the problem. Mark had what's called a varicocele, which is very common in men. A varicocele is an enlarged vein in the scrotum that causes too much blood flow to the area and decreases the quality and amount of sperm being produced. Mark's varicocele was reversed with a one-day outpatient surgery.

Yoga

Yoga is system of exercises done to attain bodily or mental control and well-being. There are different types of yoga, but all are based on ancient Hindu disciplines that promote the unity of the individual with a supreme being through a system of postures and rituals.

Yoga offers many benefits—physical, mental, and emotional, so it might be just the thing for you if you've reached a highly stressful point in your baby-making attempts.

Yoga improves muscle tone, flexibility, strength, and stamina; reduces stress and tension; boosts self-esteem; improves concentration and creativity; lowers fat; improves circulation; stimulates the immune system; and creates an overall sense of well-being and calm.

Yoga can also alleviate the symptoms of anxiety, arthritis, asthma, back pain, blood pressure, carpal tunnel syndrome, chronic fatigue, depression, diabetes, epilepsy, headaches, heart disease, multiple sclerosis, stress, and many, many other conditions and diseases.

Yoga classes are easy to find. Your local library, your community natural food store, or even your health club are good places to start.

twenty-two

Clear Your Schedule and Make Room for Baby

"**We're planning on getting** pregnant this month, and that way our children will be two years apart," Mark's colleague Jim was saying. I was overhearing Mark's conversation with his coworker.

"Yeah, right, buddy," I thought to myself, "If only it was that easy." Despite my skepticism, I was struck by the confidence and certainty in Jim's voice. There was no fear about it not happening; he just stated it as though it already was a done deal. It was a part of his child-creating process. He and his wife knew when to have sex, and that was that. Boom!—they'd be pregnant.

I remember feeling paranoid—as though he knew something I didn't—and I was dying to know how he got so darned confident about their procreation and how he sustained that energy of certainty. Listening to that conversation, I tried to contain my bitterness as I marveled at the differences between the other couple and ourselves. I longed to approach our own procreation with such certainty.

A month or so later, Mark let me know that Jim and his wife were indeed pregnant and the baby was due the coming summer. I was overwhelmed and curious as to how exactly they did it. Well, I knew *how* they did it, but I wanted to know what the difference was between them and us. They obviously had no biological concerns and approached baby-making with a totally different outlook. They just said it, and it happened. We said it, and said it, and said it—and nothing happened.

Intellectually, I knew that Mark and I had biological factors that contributed to our inability to conceive, but what came first, the chicken or the egg? Biological factors physically hinder our ability to conceive while also attacking our confidence and emotional states, which then makes it even more difficult for the physical parts to work properly. In short, hearing about Jim's success made me feel inadequate both physically and psychologically.

Just as Jim predicted, their baby came in June. By November, Mark and I had decided that we would try another IVF cycle in January. That meant we would start the process in December.

Then we were invited by a group of friends to join them on Nantucket Island for the Christmas Stroll, which always takes place the first weekend of the month. We would leave on Friday, take the high-speed ferry to the Island and eat, drink, and be merry the whole weekend through. I was looking forward to being alone with Mark and having his undivided attention.

I was also thinking that this would be our last chance to conceive naturally before again entering the high-tech world of fertility treatment. I decided to model Jim and his wife, and tried my best to have their certainty about conceiving. What a great story it would make to say that we went away for a romantic weekend and got pregnant with our baby!

"We're going to get pregnant on the Island," I announced to Mark.

Mark, the realist, wasn't buying into my plan.

"Kristen, I think that we should just expect to have a wonderful time that weekend, not expect to get pregnant. We talked about this already; we've tried for years and we need help from specialists."

"Yes, sir. Those are the facts, sir, but I want to be like Jim and his wife. I want to be in the "one enchanted evening" group and conceive a child after a wonderful date with you. So, you're going to play along with me and fake it until we make it." I was taking charge of the situation.

"So I have said, and so it shall be!" I proclaimed to myself. And put my trust in God and the Universe that we were doing the right thing. After all, we both shared the common philosophy that everything is happening the way it is supposed to, and that God has a hand in co-creating babies.

I refer to our higher power as "God," but whatever your belief system, the Universe has the ability to direct your life in the most appropriate direction. A divine directional system is what I call my "connection." For me it's just like the new cars that are equipped with a Global Positioning Satellite, which you can rely on to give you directions when necessary; your spirituality can be the connection that provides you with the strength and directions you need when navigating unknown territory.

Mark hid his concerns about my overzealous expectation for the weekend and did what every other man does in this situation: He called his mother-in-law.

A few hours later, the phone rang. It was my mom. I knew Mark had ratted me out.

"Kristen, you know we're all praying for you, but we don't want to see you get hurt again," she said.

"Mom, it's going to happen this weekend. I know it!"

I wasn't changing my approach, so Mom and Mark dropped the argument and decided to join me in my madness.

Two days before we were to leave, however, I got the stomach flu that had been going around. I felt miserable, and the thought of being on a boat at sea was not appealing. "Ma, we're not going, I feel awful. Do you guys want to go in our place?" It was a shame to let the room sit vacant.

"Oh, no, young lady, you're going! You pull yourself together, get packed, and get yourself on that island. The whole family has been praying novenas. Your aunt and I went to church all week for you. You pull yourself together and get on that boat!" My mother used her "don't mess with me" voice, so I took a deep breath, got packed, and was ready to go at the appropriate time.

The Nantucket Stroll is very charming and quite romantic. The weather was delightful and we set the course for enjoying each other while eating and drinking our way through the weekend.

To tell you the truth, I had never seen my husband as drunk as he was that Saturday night. He played the piano in the inn's living room as I'd never heard him play. His jazz renditions got our group moving and grooving, and we all were drinking like fish. At one point, Mark had to lean his head on the door jamb just to go to the bathroom. It was a first for us as a couple that one of us was that inebriated. But I couldn't blame him. I figured he needed to release the unspoken tension he felt from my high expectations of him. After all, the pres-

sure of impregnating your wife after five years of trying can send anyone on a drinking binge.

And it didn't help at all that my family kept calling to find out how
we were "doing."

"So, are you guys pregnant yet? What's taking you so long?" It was
my mom. Similar calls followed from my sister and then again from
Mom. "How's it going?" It was funny and bizarre all at the same time.
It was like a group insemination.

So, at the end of the night, with all that pressure and all that rum,
my concerns that Mark wouldn't be able to perform his manly duties
flew out of the window.

The weekend ended with a romantic ride back on the ferry, and
the month seemed to fly by. Before we knew it, the week of Christmas was upon us and, as always, my menstrual cycle was due to start
right on the holiday. I tried all month to center myself, connecting to
God and reminding myself of the certainty that I was trying to practice. I took a pregnancy test on Christmas morning, and the results
were negative. I felt different, though; but I could have been fooling
myself into interpreting all the signs of my menstrual cycle as those
of pregnancy. Nevertheless, I maintained my determined certainty,
and I felt pregnant.

Throughout Christmas Day, I began to wonder: Had I gone so far
off the deep end that I was having a hysterical pregnancy, where your
mind fools your body into thinking it's with child? Then the fear crept
in: What if it's another ectopic pregnancy that wouldn't show up on
a pregnancy test? I was slipping backward from certainty to doubt.

The next day, still with no signs of my period, Mark ran to the
local drug store where he purchased two more pregnancy tests. Wasting no time when he got back, I immediately peed on the white stick.

Holding it in my hand, we watched in awe as two purple lines appeared, indicating a positive result.

We had done it! Stunned, we embraced and I whispered, "Oh my God. We did it!" We were pregnant. Our two beautiful purple lines were later confirmed by blood work and an ultrasound, which showed a teeny sac in my uterus. The very sac that would grow over the course of the next months into our beautiful baby daughter, Grace Sarah Rose.

When Mark shared our news with his friend Jim, he told him how I had been struck by his language pattern of certainty and had tried to model his example. Jim was happy for us, of course, but surprised at how much his language about the creation of his family had affected us. Looking at Mark bewilderedly, he said, "We just knew we wanted the baby in the summer and we cleared our schedule to compensate for the growth of our family from three to four."

After a long pause, Jim asked, "Do you really think it was as simple as that?"

Mark smiled and said, "Actually, no! It's like the person who takes twenty years to become an overnight success. We've spent five years creating opportunities and experienced a lot of disappointment. As a matter of fact, we were prepared to begin IVF and we were working diligently with alternative therapies. My middle name isn't Thomas for nothing! I doubted that we could do this without medical intervention and I'm overwhelmed and in awe that we did. I guess our doctor was correct when he said that for all we know about the act of creation, there's still a lot we don't know."

So how do you clear your schedule and make room for a baby while being confronted with constant disappointment? It dawned on me that although I was practicing being mindful about having a child, speaking about it as though it *would* happen, on occasion (okay, a great deal of the time) I fell short of speaking like Mark's friend Jim, as though it were a "done deal," thus creating an opening and clearing a space for the baby without fear.

Putting It into Practice

- Managing your schedule: I encourage you to "manage your schedule" before, during, and after a fertility treatment. You have the right to decline invitations to baby showers, christenings, baby namings, or any other event. Have an "elevator speech" ready, such as, "I have a prior commitment" or "Our schedule doesn't allow us to make it." It's all about self-preservation.

- Creating a sense of certainty: How do you manage to maintain your belief that you and your partner will manifest the desired outcomes while dealing with other emotions, such as fear or doubt? After all, we are all humans here, having a human, emotional experience. For me, it boiled down to faith—believing in something without logical proof. It was natural for our friend Jim, yet unnatural for me because of our negative experiences with creation. Practice speaking or scripting your inner voice with a voice of certainty.

As Max Lucado said: "You can talk to God because God listens . . . . No need to fear that you will be ignored. Even if you stammer or stumble, even if what you have to say impresses no one, it impresses God—and He listens."

twenty-three

Keeping Love on the Rocks

It was 5:15 Friday afternoon, and I was eager to call it the official start of the weekend. But my e-mail icon was blinking, so I reluctantly opened my inbox and began to scan my messages. Serendipitously, one e-mail contained a gift. Once again, the universe had brought me an opportunity for growth.

The e-mail was from a close friend, just sending me some news and a brief update. She closed by saying that she was running off to the video store after work to pick up a new release and that she anticipated having Chinese food, watching the movie, and having a home date with her husband.

I marveled at this for two reasons: (1) she was up on the current trend of movie releases; and (2) she planned a home date with her husband.

My friend is the sort of woman who has her life planned to the point of knowing what she and her husband will be doing for work and recreation the entire month. She is so focused and accomplishes so much, she often makes Mark and me feel like we're lazy bums—and we work hard enough! (This is a woman who has a standing appointment with her stylist every six weeks. I, on the other hand, wait for my hair to be hanging in my eyes, and then call my hairdresser in a panic because my hair looks like a mop.) And here she was, planning, as usual, a delightful evening for herself and her husband.

It made me stop and think: How could I be so attentive and organized for work, but so disorganized in the recreational side of our life?

Mark and I worked hard and had goals and objectives that took a great deal of our attention. Then, come Saturday, we were totally unprepared for downtime. We would wake up in the morning and allow the day to slip away, then try to plan a fun activity by the seat of our pants. Don't get me wrong, being spontaneous is exciting, but for us it didn't exactly work. It seemed as though we were a dog chasing its tail and ending up in circles:

"What do you want to do?"

"I dunno. What do you want to do?"

Around and around we would go, moving no closer to fun than a dog moving closer to its tail!

I became motivated to model the spirit of organized fun in my friend's e-mail, and decided to create the same system for our household.

Mark and I had stopped paying attention to play time, especially when consumed with creating our family. We were taskmasters moving forward on completing our work without sustaining a sense of relaxation or balance in our relationship. What we needed to do was to put just as much focus on play as we did on work.

Filling the Jar

Stephen Covey, author of *The 7 Habits of Highly Effective People,* uses a remarkable exercise in his seminars. Dr. Covey uses a glass jar to represent life, and large and small rocks to represent life's priorities. On the largest rocks, he writes the words "love," "family," "religion," etc. His point is that life can be made up of many things, not just your priorities. He demonstrates his point by first placing the large "priority" rocks into the empty jar. Then he pours sand over the rocks, filling the jar to the tiptop while asking, "Is it full yet?" He then quietly pours water into the jar. It's a great visual that demonstrates how important it is to put the priority rocks of your life in the jar first, because only then will the sand and water of your life fill in around the cracks.

The process of creating our family took center stage in our activities. It seemed as though our attention went in patterns. We'd go through a phase where we were great at maintaining focus on our relationship and planning long weekends, dates, and special nights with friends and family, but then life seemed to take over and unplanned events unfolded, sucking our attention away from our core. Our dates were either canceled or postponed and never completed. Just like a clock pendulum, our relationship would swing to a priority position and then slowly begin to swing out of view.

Mark and I needed to empty out our relationship jar and begin to fill it in with us *first*. The most prominent rock had to be our relationship rock and all that it represents: procreation, love, creativity, alone time, and together time. Then—and only then—could we add in all the other responsibilities and aspects of our life—work, our house, and our families.

We both knew about the jar and all that it represented; we had simply forgotten. That Friday afternoon, I was grateful that my friend's e-mail had "jarred" my memory.

Before Mark got home, I decided to write down how I thought we could recreate our own loving jar. So with day-runner and calendar in hand, I started. I determined that we'd have dinner together three times a week and would schedule a surprise date night for each other once a month. The date night would consist of something we'd been wanting to do and the other party would have to play along with what was preordained. I plugged in some dates and began to work outward to the next month to give us a few opportunities to make sure this renewed "rock in the jar" concept took hold once again.

I was sure that the jar was the answer to how we could keep our marriage centered and in balance, not swinging from side to side—attended versus neglected.

Mark was very receptive to our new plan of scheduled recreational activities and focusing on all parts of our life. He added a few terrific comments and suggestions to the list I had prepared.

That Saturday, Mark and I found a clean glass jar. We found a smooth rock that would fit into the opening. I wrote "love" on the face of the rock with an indelible marker and gently placed it into the jar. We followed it with other, smaller stones, also marked with meaningful priorities. We filled around the stones with sand and then topped off the jar with water. Although our priorities shift periodically, we keep that jar on our shelf.

Our love is still on the rocks and our jar runneth over.

Putting It into Practice

Using the glass jar analogy, fill *your* life's jar! First with rocks, which represent the most important parts of your life, then with sand, which fills in around the rocks, and finally with water, making your life complete. When we were in baby-creating mode, there were only two rocks in our jar, work and baby; it was the simple act of planning recreation that brought us to the point of having a full relationship.

❀ Start by jotting down all the words that represent the important parts of your life. You might want to actually do the exercise, attaching them to a rock and placing them into a glass jar. It's a great exercise for a visual person. Some of our other words were relationship, together time, religion, and family.

❀ Then jot down words that represent what is important but not the main focus of your life. These words will be represented by sand and gravel. Take a moment and think as you move one consecutive circle out from the most important aspects of your lives. What would the grains of sand be?

❀ Don't forget water! The water represents more of the mundane responsibilities that we all have to do. Pushing yet one more circle out from the most important part or core of your life, how will you see the liquid part of the glass jar? Paying bills, going grocery shopping, mowing the lawn?

❀ Make a plan for how you and your partner are going to arrange your life so that the most important aspects, the rocks, become the focus of your life and relationship. It's a physical representation of a game plan, and will help you create a foundation that is truly important.

❀ Remind yourself that a relationship is work, and that you must give it attention and care each and every day. This can be achieved by planning recreational activities. Biweekly or monthly events, something to look forward to together, can bring some fun anticipation into your days, and bring you closer as a couple.

It's Okay to Take a Time-Out

As I was heading up the stairs toward our bedroom I realized that old saying, "never go to bed angry" wasn't working in our household. It wasn't that we were "mad" at each other, we hadn't had a misunderstanding or a heated discussion, but it was obvious the energy between us was just . . . prickly.

Mark was visibly tired and a bit cranky, having just arrived home from an eight-day business trip. I know that when he travels his schedule is brutal: waiting in the airport for flights that are delayed more often than not, arriving late at his destination, and waking early to present his seminar from 7:00 AM to 6:00 PM, with no chance for exercise or downtime. Exercise is a significant factor in Mark's constitution, and if he doesn't run he's not that pleasant to be around.

Still, I couldn't help but think about the glamorous side of business travel. In my view, when you're traveling, you have work responsibilities to focus your attention on, and that's about it. There is no laundry to be done, no trash to be dragged out, no bills to be paid, or grocery shopping to be done. It's pretty much your work, eating dinner out in a restaurant, and having your breakfast delivered to you in your room on a heated plate. It has an allure to me.

After all, when Mark's away, I'm a single working woman with all the responsibilities. On top of my own work, I have all the responsibilities of our home life on my shoulders. I've found it's not the large responsibilities that take their toll when you're a single working person; it's the small stuff. Like when the dryer breaks mid-load or the outdoor lamp light burns out and it's ten below zero outside.

Admittedly, the scenario of Mark having the sweeter end of the deal while he traveled was pure projection on my part and probably very far from the truth, but that's how I viewed what had transpired over the course of the last eight days.

Left out of the glamorous travel scene I had conjured in my head was the fact that Mark booked his out-of-town work engagements around my menstrual cycle, in order to be home at the appropriate time for procreation. That the brunt of our finances is on his shoulders and he continually meets that responsibility; that he is a thoughtful, warm-hearted person who loves me dearly—this all gets tossed aside as I scan for evidence that supports my position.

So how do you put aside all those emotions that contribute to the prickly, unhealthy feelings? How do you cope with all the normal marital emotions and move through them to get down to the business at hand—procreation?

Remember "time-outs" from kindergarten?

When I ran a day care center, I was surrounded by fifty-one children every day. We had a non-violence school philosophy that was strictly enforced through time-outs. If there was a conflict between two five-year-olds that couldn't be resolved, I called a time-out, and each child was given a special chair to sit in for a few minutes to ponder a solution. The time-out never once failed to work. That brief cooling-down period provided a time for each child to regroup and assess the situation. And it provided me an opportunity to teach numerous lessons on interpersonal relationships.

So by heading up those stairs to our bedroom this night, it wasn't so much that I was going to bed "mad. " In truth, I was employing the time-out concept—and it seemed to be working. I was giving myself a chance to regroup and realize that whatever Mark was thinking or feeling really had nothing to do with me, and I couldn't take it personally. I dropped the "celebrity" status that I had given Mark's role of making our life work financially and reminded myself that we're in this together.

I decided to give Mark as much emotional slack as I had when we were first dating. You know what I mean: that point in your relationship when you're so deeply in love that if your partner told you he'd just wrecked your car, you'd say, "That's okay, I was thinking about getting a new one anyway." It seemed that no matter what he or she did, the romance goggles allowed you to view the behavior as appropriate, wonderful, and even sexy! So that's what I would do with Mark. I'd put on my romance goggles and treat him as though we just started out in our relationship, not that we were ten years into it and burping at the dinner table was as common as passing the salt.

At the end of my time-out, I shook off those envious feelings, took a deep breath, and headed down the stairs to find Mark.

Putting It into Practice

1. Take a time-out. At one time or another, I believe every couple has experienced those "prickly" feelings in their relationship, and, in my book, a time-out is the best way to clear the air. Physically moving out of each other's energy and personal space can do wonders for your emotional health and rejuvenate your feelings toward your partner.

2. Pause and regroup. Take a moment to calm down and breathe deeply for a few seconds. It will work wonders for your body and relieve the adrenaline that is flowing though your bloodstream.

3. Assess the situation. As difficult as it may be, emotionally remove yourself from the battle and try not to take everything personally. This is a marriage-saver! It all goes back to being loving even though your fight-or-flight response is kicking in to protect you from a perceived threat or attack. By taking a time-out, you can disengage from the negative energy poisoning your relationship and view your situation from a healthier, more positive perspective.

4. Find the lesson. Rather than dwelling on the negative, try to view your disagreements as chances to learn how to resolve your interpersonal conflicts more quickly and easily. After all, what would be the point of these exchanges if they weren't opportunities for growth? Just take an emotional breather, move past the ugly stuff, and find the lesson.

5. Put on your romance goggles. Try to get back to the earlier "dates" of your relationship in your mind's eye and bring back those romantic, he-or she-can-do-no-wrong feelings. Earlier, in Strategy Six, I talked about writing your love story on the first page of your journal to remember why you fell in love with your partner, to reconnect with your romantic feelings. Well, the romance goggles strategy works along the same lines, but is used during a marital time-out. All couples encounter marital hurdles, but when a relationship is compounded by the intense emotional weight of trying to create a baby, the need for this strategy is even greater. To rediscover those loving goggles, just remember an awesome date from your romantic past and connect with that time or date emotionally to reclaim your connecion. This little visit to the past will help remove the marital warts of the present.

twenty-five

Pamper Your Mind, Body, and Soul

The bubbles of the foot spa swirled around my ankles as I sat in the vibrating, heated chair. I wasn't used to having my hands and feet touched, and as much as I tried to relax, I still was holding tension in my fingers and toes.

Upon the insistence of my best friend, Rosie, I was having my first manicure and pedicure.

"I'm coming to take you for a pedicure and manicure; you've been looking like hell lately and it's time you put some attention back on yourself and grow up and expose your toes," Rosie's voice had barked at me that morning.

She had watched my personality change dramatically from the strain of fertility treatments and had planned this spa visit as part of a girls-only outing.

The technician had a ready smile and maneuvered through the pedicure with ease. I felt like a fish out of water, totally unaware of the "salon" protocol. This outing was supposed to be a chance to be pampered but, as I glanced down at my feet, all I really felt was embarrassment. I never really liked the way my toes looked and hid them most of the time in sneakers, shying away from open-toed sandals.

"So, whaddaya think?" Rosie asked as we left the salon.

Looking down at my toes and fingers, freshly painted in a bright "Saucy Salsa" red, I said, "I don't know. It was okay—my feet aren't that much of an embarrassment. Thanks for making me go, Rosie. You're a good woman."

I drove home, admiring the flashes of red that caught my eye as I steered or adjusted the radio station. Then, out of the blue, I began to cry. Life had been difficult for the past few months, with disappointing results from our procreation efforts, and I appreciated Rosie pulling me out of my comfort zone and into the salon.

This trip to the salon represented something other than a girls' outing. It was a screaming reminder that I had yet another part of my life out of balance. The fact was that, through all the months spent hoping and praying for a baby, I neglected my other female side—the side of me that took pride in maintaining my appearance, that wore makeup and dressed in clothes that actually matched. It had been a slow and steady slide down to where I no longer cared about my appearance. All I cared about was getting pregnant. Pulling myself together as I drove up our driveway, I was careful not to mar my still-wet polish. I ran up to Mark and proudly displayed my hands and feet.

"Wow! That looks great—and quite sexy. Why don't you do that more often?" he said, kissing my hand while winking.

Hmmm. My painted nails had triggered something in Mark! He was connecting my sexy toes with sex! How, I'm not really sure. But I thought I would go with this, since we had viewed sex as only one thing for so long: an activity to produce an offspring.

I would never have thought that a little glass jar of red nail polish could ignite a flash of passion in our relationship. But it did. The simple act of painting my nails nurtured both our sexual relationship and the truly feminine side of me.

I determined right then and there that I would come up with a strategy to keep my feminine side thriving and nurtured while, at the same time, enduring all that was necessary to create a family.

Then out of the blue I remembered a conversation I had once had with Dr. Ali Domar, who wrote a book on self-nurturing titled *Self-Nurture: Learning to Care for Yourself as Effectively as You Care for Everyone Else.* During our conversation, she told me, "It's so important to learn to self-nurture before you have children and make it a priority, because after you have children you won't have time."

As the light bulb went off over my head, my jaw dropped. And it dawned on me: Self-nurturing is a *learned* behavior for women.

I had never considered my craniosacral appointment a form of pampering or self-nurturing, but in light of my nail-painting revelations, I realized that it was. I wasn't totally ignoring that part of me; that part was getting some of its needs met when I took the time and worked with Lisa, my wonderful therapist. It wasn't until the pedicure that I realized that I was viewing my craniosacral appointments as "work" and totally blanked on the fact that it fell into the self-nurturing category as well. Suddenly, the light bulb went on again, and I realized that all my other strategies, such as journaling, yoga, and meditation, were actually forms of self-nurturing, too. It had been all work to me; just another means of coping with our infertility issues rather than exercises to benefit my mind, body, and soul.

I think this false association originated from my Catholic upbringing, which instilled in me a sense of guilt about enjoying pleasure.

With this subconscious belief that taking time for myself was being selfish, I had an underlying need to make an "excuse" for my craniosacral therapy appointments, to justify the treatments under the banner of infertility therapy.

But it was time for me to shake off the guilt and celebrate all the facets of my being—mind, body, and soul—and learn how to care for each. I would be a better woman—and mother —for it.

With that subtle shift of thinking, my appointments with Lisa took on a different meaning, and I began a new ritual. On the drive to the appointments, I began giving thanks for the opportunity to nurture my mind, body, and soul. I allowed myself to acknowledge the dual purpose of our meetings and gave myself permission to embrace the experience as self-nurturing.

That was years ago. Now both Mark and I fully embrace our favorite means of "pampering." For Mark, it's a massage, and for me, it's my biweekly craniosacral treatments. For those brief sixty minutes, I thrive; I allow my mind, body, and soul to be cleansed, regenerated, and—most importantly—pampered.

Putting It into Practice

1. Give yourself permission to be self-nurturing. It's easy to be overwhelmed by the emotional, physical, and spiritual demands of fertility treatments, not to mention the hectic schedule. So the first step is to remind yourself that you must care for all parts of your being during this time and embrace the idea of pampering yourself. Sit for a moment and think of how your body, mind, and soul might react to being self-nurtured. Envision what might be the best form of self-nurturing for you.

2. Make a list. Take a moment and think about what you are already doing, and give yourself credit for self-nurturing. If you implemented any of the strategies shared in this book, you can put them under the self-nurturing category. On a piece of paper, jot down five things that you think could be your own private self-nurturing treat. Choose something that doesn't require a huge effort, something that you can fit into your ritual once a day or once a week, whichever you feel more comfortable with. That way, you'll be more apt to stick with it. Remember, your self-nurturing doesn't have to be extravagant; it could be a hot cup of tea, a conversation with a friend, a manicure, an exercise routine, a hot shower or bath, or a quick trip to your favorite store. As the saying goes, it's the little things that count. (My sister, a hospital nurse, admitted that every day, after lunch, she treats herself to five cents' worth of penny candy at the gift shop. It's her little indulgence in her rather hectic life, but that's all she needs.)

What can you do daily (and stick with it), that will make you feel pampered and special?

Making Love vs. Making Work

"**I want to go out to lunch!** I want to wear sandals! And where's all the condos they promised?" There I stood with a dripping paint roller in hand, trying to imitate Goldie Hawn's role in *Private Benjamin*.

Mark took a momentary break from the wall he was painting in our living room and gave me a "don't start with that again" look.

I'd gotten bids to have professionals paint our two rooms, but that frugal—okay, cheap—part of me cringed at the prices. We could do it ourselves, I thought, and save the money for the new furniture we wanted.

"We *can* afford to have this done professionally, Kristen, and then save to buy the furniture," Mark had reminded me. But I just couldn't bring myself to write that check.

"Come on, it'll be fun!" I crooned to Mark. By using his pleasure-seeking language pattern as a form of enticement, I thought I could sweeten the pot.

He agreed and on a fall Saturday morning, we began our attack. Not long into our work, I realized that the color I'd chosen—or perhaps it was my painting technique—wasn't looking as good as I had hoped.

Then I looked over at Mark's side of the room, and things were looking better.

"Boy, you're doing a great job over there; your painting experience is really showing through. Was it for two or three summers that you worked as a house painter?" I grinned.

There was no response from Mark. He just continued to face his wall and rolled two more roller lengths. I could almost see the "I told you so" being worked out through the pressure he exerted into his roller. By that afternoon, the two rooms looked great. "It almost looks professionally done!" Mark said excitedly. Then I understood—all along, he was concerned that the results would not be up to par.

"It sure does! Maybe we have a new business endeavor staring us in the face?" I really was joking.

"Go get your sandals. I'll take you out for a late lunch." Mark headed to the kitchen to wash the painting supplies.

"Yippee, another job well done!" I screamed, racing up to the shower.

While in our shower, scrubbing off the remnants of the khaki green paint, I realized that by sharing the time to paint our rooms, I felt quite intimate with Mark. Who knew that through working together we would find a connection that was normally gained through sexual intimacy? Especially considering that our current lovemaking was work, as in scheduled, timed, and documented in a medical record.

But right then, both of us clean and dewy from the shower, we started getting frisky, and . . . I'll just say we had a later lunch than we'd planned on. . . .

Lost sexual intimacy had been the prime topic of numerous exchanges in our marriage. The type-A girl knew that, to achieve pregnancy, abstinence a few days prior to the "most fertile" days would make for a better sperm deposit from Mark, and that having sexual intercourse every other day during the most fertile phase would increase our odds. Therefore, with calendars in hand, we broke the month down into thirds: the first third was a free time, while the second third was critical and very regimented, but the last third of the month, there was really no reason to have sex because "procreation time" had passed. The last third was officially the waiting period, fraught with all the emotions that came with waiting for a positive pregnancy test. Who really needed sex at that point?

It was so mechanical and so business-like.

Yet those measures are wildly passionate compared with the cold, regimented territory of the high-tech fertility world, where not only is your most private act regulated by your hormonally induced cycle, but you now have a whole team of people governing all your sexual activity. Out the window flew any sense of normalcy, and in the door came a strained, robotic marriage.

How can you manage any sense of intimacy while dealing with the business of making a baby?

For us, the answer presented itself through a work strategy: negotiation.

We were refining our negotiating skills through our many business transactions with our clients, using the common phrase "Is this a deal-maker?" to identify the most important issues to each party. There would be times when we both wanted to have sex, but because of where we were on our fertility cycle, it was best that we didn't. So we agreed to use the "deal-maker" rationale when scheduling sex to ensure our sexual needs would be met.

We would pencil in unbridled, toe-curling sex along with quickies and specialized individual attention when necessary. This "negotiation" totally stripped (no pun intended) the romance and spontaneity out of our sexual relationship, but at least we would know where the other person stood and we could attempt to meet each other's needs. Is it possible to schedule romance and spontaneity?

Then I heard an interview with Dr. John Gray (author of *Men Are From Mars, Women Are From Venus*) on the radio. Dr. Gray shared his view that a woman's sex drive is like a Crock-Pot, a slow-cooker that takes a while to heat up to the appropriate temperature but, as soon as the pot is up to the right degree, the meal is ready—and look out! The male, on the other hand, is a microwave; enough said. For women, what counts is the quality of the relationship, the connection between her partner and herself, and having the time necessary to achieve sexual pleasure. For men, it's not necessary to "feel" anything to have sex.

Dr. Gray was addressing the "normal" male/female relationship, and noted that the average couple has sexual intercourse two times a week.

Normal? Average? We'd been trying to have a baby for three years! And with our work schedules, sometimes Mark and I didn't even have time to have dinner together two times a week, never mind making love.

I began accepting that we would need to work on our sexual relationship to keep some fire burning. After all, a good relationship just doesn't happen; it requires careful attention and work each and every day. And sex is part of every good relationship, so creating a ritual to meet each other's sexual needs before we have a family, during good times and bad, would make the transition from married people having sex to married *parents* having sex less complicated.

Instead of viewing our newly designed ritual as work, I decided to view it as a sexual insurance policy—insuring that we would communicate our needs, schedule our "appointments," and reap the benefits of the emotional connection that comes with good lovemaking. A definite win-win all around!

Putting It into Practice

1. Get together. Share what is important for you to feel connected sexually. Mark and I actually found that this was easier than anticipated. Mark needed to know that he was going to have a special sexual night, guaranteed regardless of life's interruptions. He also negotiated "dinner and a movie" each month; it could be out for a movie or a home movie night that ended with sex. Those were his deal-makers. I called my deal the "Private Benjamin." The evening would be completed with a sexual experience that started with long kisses and progressed to the promised land. It would be great if this could occur during prime baby-making time so that "one enchanted evening" group need would be fulfilled.

2. Make a deal. As in any good negotiation, if you give something, you have to get something in return. With that in mind, I was willing to negotiate for one over-the-edge evening and one middle-of-the-road planned "date," which became our "Thursday Breakfast" date. Because of Mark's schedule, the weekends were often interrupted and, on some occasions, our weekend was during the middle of the week. Thursday morning became our date morning. We would go out for breakfast, come home to have alone time, and then go to work. This schedule worked wonderfully for us because we worked together and could arrange our schedules. The breakfast date kept that connection alive and well during all of the infertility stresses and the pressures of everyday life. I needed that!

3. Create an ironclad termination policy. Make your plans for intimacy the highest priority between you. This agreement is not to be broken, but if an extreme situation arises, you can reschedule for another day or night. We stuck to the ironclad policy and reaped benefits beyond the obvious physical ones—subconscious benefits from the knowledge that the importance of our intimacy outweighed all of life's other demands. Your time together is crucial, and these dates are a done deal. Remember your rocks in the jar.

twenty-seven

Listen for Your Inner Voice

Payday at Cricket's Corner Learning Center was on Thursdays. While a joyous day for my employees, payday was the most stressful part of managing my company.

When I opened the school, I was still wet behind the ears when it came to the workings of payroll and the taxes that were due to the Internal Revenue Service each quarter. My biggest responsibilities were to my staff—to ensure they did get paid on Thursdays—and also to the state and federal government, to ensure timely payments of the huge tax bills, which would earn late penalties if deposited after the fifteenth of the month. For years, my greatest fear was that one week I would not be able to meet my payroll.

Then one week my fear came true. It was Tuesday and, in two days, I would have to write checks for thousands of dollars and make additional deposits to the government for thousands more, but—according to my checkbook—I was short. Panic set in; I plopped myself onto the sofa in my office, and put my face in my hands in an attempt to hide my tears. From out of nowhere came a strange sense of certainty. With my eyes closed, a mental movie began to play. In the movie, I was at the front door of the school, walking back to my office while flipping through that day's mail. Among the envelopes in my hand was the substantial check I had been waiting for to relieve my financial pressure.

When the "daydream" was over, I opened my eyes and dried my tears. I had to refocus my thoughts at least until later in the day when the mail came.

With that game plan in mind, I went about my morning routine with the children, then headed for the front door to greet the mailman, who arrived right on time with a fat stack of mail.

Heading back to my office, shuffling through the envelopes, my eyes landed on the envelope that held the substantial payment. My feelings and prior daydream became real, and with relief I met my payroll responsibilities to all parties that week.

At the time, I didn't really grasp the whole meaning behind what had happened that morning in my office. I did realize that I felt different and received information through my daydream, but I dismissed the possibility that there might be a connection between being in a stressful situation and looking inward for guidance. Then, on that Tuesday, the light bulb finally turned on. I had been terrified of not being able to meet my financial responsibilities, and the fear created tension and stress, which was both emotionally and physically damaging. With my stern inner voice I talked to myself: "Kristen, you've always met your responsibilities; God and the Universe have always sent you the money necessary. Why in the world are you discounting the feelings of certainty and replacing them with doubt? Trust the knowing part of you and the Universe."

So what was that glimpse into the future and that sudden feeling of certainty?

My intuition.

Intuition is a sense of knowing about a given situation without actually having concrete evidence or facts to support it. Throughout most of my life, however, I had been hearing from my intuition, but not truly *listening* to it. Tapping into your own intuition can be intimidating. Intuition is a powerful tool that we all possess. The ability to connect to this "internal guidance system," like the global positioning system we use on our boat, took practice.

Let's go back to Strategy Ten, where you identified your and your partner's individual communication strategies as either visual, auditory, or kinesthetic. You can also use this technique to discover how you connect with your intuitive sense and receive information. If, for example, your score revealed that you're auditory, your intuition might come as a voice or sound in your head. If you are visually oriented, you might see a glimpse of the future in a daydream or night dream. Whereas, if you are a feeling-oriented person, you might have a gut feeling or a feeling of heaviness when trying to make a decision that could be interpreted as a sign to slow down prior to coming to a conclusion.

Have you ever walked into a room filled with people and been drawn to a certain person, having an instant energetic connection or a sense that you had met somewhere before? Or perhaps during a business or personal meeting you had a strong gut feeling that a topic being proposed wasn't going to work out? It could have been a feeling or hearing something or maybe even seeing something in the way the information was presented, but it all comes from a sense of knowing. If you followed those clues, did the situation play out in the manner that you foresaw?

I began to learn more about intuition by reading books and attending seminars. I even had meetings with two women who are intuitive consultants in an attempt to help us through our procreation journey. Then I began sharing my findings with Mark, who was not at all tuned in to his intuition. As a very focused businessman, he was in the practice of relying on facts and concrete evidence to make a decision, but facts alone are not enough. In light of my research, he began trying to connect on a more regular basis with his own intuition. It felt strange to him at the beginning, just as it did with me. As it is said, practice makes perfect, but in this case practice makes the feeling more acceptable.

Let me share with you two examples of how Mark and I relied on our intuition to guide us in making the right choices for us when it came to addressing our infertility.

At the beginning of our creation journey, I had a sense that something wasn't quite right, a strong sense that we needed medical intervention. I had no credible evidence to support these feelings, but they would just appear to me as a sense of doubt about our ability to conceive. With that sense, I fudged the time that we had been having unprotected intercourse (a year) and made an appointment with an obstetrician/gynecologist after only eight months of trying.

At our first meeting, I had some negative feelings about the doctor and the way we were relating. An inner voice seemed to be shouting that he wasn't a match for me, but I stifled that little voice and continued under his care for quite some time. Longer than I should have, as it turns out, because my intuition was correct. He was an obstetrician and a gynecologist, not a reproductive endocrinologist. After several months under his care, and still no result, I finally listened to my inner voice.

Even though I wasn't sure where to get help or who to turn to, my intuition had been trying to steer me in the right direction.

Finally listening to that part and taking action brought us to the correct doctor; we found "Dr. Right," and immediately I felt safe with him and knew he would help us. Sure enough, when we began our initial fertility work, we decided that surgery was necessary for me. When facing surgery, I "checked in" with my intuition and felt that it was okay to go ahead with the surgery.

After the surgery, three cycles of intrauterine insemination, an ectopic pregnancy, and my bout with a deep depression, we had another meeting with "Dr. Right" to create another game plan. The outcome of that meeting was that we should enter into a cycle of IVF.

Upon hearing this, I just could not bring myself to accept this next step. I was exhausted and seemed to have no energy to get through my days. Whenever I asked myself the question, "Should we start an IVF cycle now?" I saw a stop sign. It was big and red and screaming, "STOP!" Once again, I had no concrete evidence to explain why we shouldn't begin IVF, but I listened to my inner voice and waited until I felt comfortable about a starting date before making an appointment. When I told the doctor about my hesitation to start IVF again, he did a blood test, which revealed that I was anemic and explained why I'd been feeling so tired. Mark and I agreed to wait for my body to recover and my anemia to improve before beginning the IVF. "Checking in" with our intuition proved to be a valuable tool.

Putting It into Practice

1. Use your voice. Give voice to and acknowledge the information that you are receiving, be it through a feeling, a picture, or a message in your mind. Identify your feelings and explain them to yourself and/or your partner. For example, "I am feeling a heaviness about the prospect of having surgery."

2. Ask why. Ask yourself a question about the feeling: "Why am I feeling this heaviness?" or, "Should I proceed with the surgery?"

3. Sense. Sit quietly and wait for information to come through a feeling, a vision, or a voice in your head. Be aware of all your senses. If information doesn't present itself right away, make a conscious decision to give in to that knowing part of yourself and release the question. Maybe you are unable to connect right at the moment, especially when stress is involved. It's all right. Just check in again—making sure to ask the same question when you do.

4. Interpret. What is your intuition telling you? Is it guiding you to a positive or a mental image or feeling? Once again using the surgery example, when I did the above three steps, the information I received was through a mental movie and a feeling. I saw myself in a hospital gown coming out of the anesthesia and I was fine. I interpreted the information received as a feeling of peace and well-being. I then knew it was right for me to have surgery.

5. Practice. If at first you don't succeed, try, try again! This whole process should only take a few moments. For some of you, this strategy might be a stretch outside of your traditional comfort zone. But tapping into your intuition is like turning on the VCR: You have to keep your television on either channel 3 or 4 in order to play the tape. It's the same for tuning into your intuition; you have to be on the right channel or wavelength to receive the signs to play!

And just like your television, sometimes you have to fiddle with the antenna to get good reception. Keep working at your intuition and eventually the picture will be crystal clear!

twenty-eight

Celebrate Victories

The gratitude principle, in a nutshell, states that when you stop feeling gratitude, you stop progressing, either at work or at home. Dan Sullivan, Mark's strategic coach, came to this understanding during his twenty years of working with a variety of people. He concluded that the level of gratitude you hold is in direct correlation to your success and your level of upward mobility. "To explain the principle," Mark told me, "Sullivan used the example of a man who was a great success, but had lost the connection to the people who had helped him create his life. He thought he could do it all alone. Subsequently, with this lack of gratitude for his supporters, he was getting a divorce and his business was in a steep decline."

I'm pretty confident that all the time Mark was listening to Dan's story, he was changing the names and events to correlate with our situation. Mark blamed our gradual loss of connection on the dwindling amount of abundance in our lives, fearing that our future contained only further decline.

Ironically, only an hour earlier, I had been the person so empty of gratitude. Just that afternoon, I had been sitting on our front steps telling my close friend Sarah how upset I was that a family member was going to have another child. The news of their new baby reopened the wounds of our difficulty having a family. As I sat there crying, Sarah listened attentively and compassionately, all the while providing a grounding voice, which brought me back to my true reality: I had a blessed life.

"Kristen, I know that hearing news of the pregnancy sent you for a loop, and it's okay to feel that way," she said, first acknowledging where I was on the emotional-wreck-meter, then she hugged me and continued. "You and Mark have a wonderful life, Kristen. You're so blessed. I admire your dedication to helping others and your ability to do it all. And you brighten people's lives, especially mine." She gave me final tight squeeze and ran to retrieve her own son from the school bus.

Hearing the "we're having a baby" news again from my relative made me feel as though I was living on an island surrounded by women who could get pregnant at the drop of a coconut. I allowed feelings of isolation, despair, and sadness to take over, and held onto them tightly.

Then as I watched Sarah quickly run across the front yard, I was so upset with myself for the lack of gratitude I showed. Sarah was so right; I was living a blessed life with my family and friends, and the work successes I'd achieved. When was the last time I had thanked Sarah for her friendship? When was the last time I had told Mark how much I appreciated him, for that matter? Even though I expressed my gratitude for them nightly in my journal, it was a private form of giving thanks; I was failing at telling them and others how grateful I was for them in my life. I was the man in Dan Sullivan's story. I had lost my focus on expressing thanks and on celebrating the victories of each day.

Sarah had taught me that you needed to celebrate your victories, not wallow in your failures. We often talked, and Sarah consistently set an obtainable goal for herself daily. At the end of the day, she felt victorious about completing that goal. She was always grateful and celebratory.

I tried to model her behavior and that same sense of celebration of life and gratitude for each day. But, being confronted with our baby-creating challenges, I drifted away from that spirit. Strategy Twenty-eight explores the impact gratitude can have on the process of creation and introduces the concept of recognizing moments of gratitude. Creating these moments helps you focus on the good things in your life and lets you tune out the unproductive negative chatter that some of our unhealthy emotions can produce. This strategy has proven helpful for many of us facing the procreation challenge.

For celebrating victories, gratitude plays a different role. In this context, gratitude is key to developing a habit of celebration and needs to be consistently woven into the fabric of your daily life. With that in mind, I'd like to share with you two examples of how my family started to celebrate minor daily events. Remember the Honey-Do List in Strategy Seventeen? How Mark wanted an official after-work greeting daily? I made it my goal to give Mark that two-second greeting, and in my mind I transformed it into one of my celebrations of the day. After spending the day apart and completing our individual responsibilities, we celebrate our reunion and safe return home at the end of the day. This welcoming celebration has become an important part of our lives; our five-year-old son, who now participates in this evening ritual, views this as "normal."

Another example of simple acts of celebration is giving thanks at the beginning of your dinner. Gratitude here, for us, stems from the spiritual concept of thanking the Universe and God for the wonderful food we will be eating and to celebrate the efforts it took to bring that food onto the table. Our dinnertime blessing was also a forum for non-culinary statements of gratitude. For example, while I was writing this book, every night at the dinner celebration my son would say, ". . . and thank you for Mom almost completing her book." His thankfulness changed the context of my daily struggles. With that expression of abundance, he helped me transform the stress of writing a book into a wonderful challenge that I was blessed to experience.

Applying the same philosophy to fertility, we can all be thankful for the amazing technological breakthroughs of the past several years—for the opportunity to make our baby-creating dreams become reality, no matter what the odds.

Putting It into Practice

1. Celebrate even the tiny victories. When heartbreaking news arrives, and your fragile dream of parenthood falls from its pedestal and shatters into a million pieces, it can be hard enough not to spend the whole day crying, let alone find something to be grateful for. But there's always something to celebrate. Are you otherwise healthy? Be grateful. Did you meet your goals for the day? Be grateful. Did you make it to the gas station on fumes, without running out of gas? Celebrate! That's a victory. Look for that tiny speck to cling to in your current situation.

2. Create the habit. Take a moment and look at your daily life. Is there a time during the day that you can integrate a celebration? After we've eaten dinner and cleaned up the dishes, we crank up Cher's song "Believe" and sing at the top of our lungs, dancing around like hotties from the seventies. We look forward to that moment, as it reminds us to believe in life's opportunities. What I didn't realize is that you can see into our kitchen from the street, and one night I arrived home after dinner and, passing our house to pull into our driveway, I could see Mark and Cole dancing away. From the outside looking in, it looked like complete mania, but I knew what was happening, and it warmed my heart.

What little ritual can you create that would have its own secret meaning, puzzling to someone looking in from the outside?

3. Don't diminish your achievements. One of the experiential programs we offer in our seminars is the "Firewalk Experience," where participants walk over 1200-degree coals that we make by burning oak to red-hot embers. During the seminar, we help people look at their fears and use some of the strategies I've shared with you in this book to take action and overcome them. It's amazing to me that after the participants visit the fire and are assured that it is real, feeling the searing heat on their legs, they willingly walk the intimidating eight-foot path.

For me, the Firewalk is a perfect metaphor for infertility. When I walked the walk, feeling the heat on a few occasions, I would lose my focus and want to jump off the path. But I didn't. I would regain my composure and stay focused on my goal of getting to the other side.

How easy it is for us humans to face extraordinary challenges when we really put our minds to it! Like the participants in our Firewalk, you can overcome your fears and diminish your obstacles by persevering through the emotional, physical, and spiritual challenges you are working through to create your family.

Take a moment to make a list of all you've gone through in pursuit of your dreams. Acknowledge your own personal Firewalk, then celebrate it.

4. Don't forget that you're not alone. When facing infertility, you may feel as though you are the only person or couple experiencing this heartbreak. But, unfortunately, you're not. One in six couples cannot create their baby as they had envisioned. The one thing I wish I had done differently was to attend support groups and more workshops. We found the support through RESOLVE well into our journey. I encourage you to join your local chapter of RESOLVE or a similar organization such as AIA (American Infertility Association). After we joined, I devoured the newsletter and then began to attend workshops. I was truly thankful that I did. Always remember: You are not alone.

In closing, I'd like to share with you one of my favorite poems my friend Sarah shared with me:

How to Live on an Island
by Sandy Gingras*

Dance on edges, stretch, listen in on shells, put living things back,
Cultivate quiet, boogie, practice simplicity, sugar yourself with sand,
Float, carry a bucket, ride rusty bikes—go with the wind, walk tender, respect
Leave no wake, tune up your senses, build castles and leave them for the moon to find,
Run with waves, discover treasure, remember yourself, keep off the rocks, ebb and flow
Laugh like a gull, thank.

*Reprinted, with permission, from the book, *How to Live on an Island,* by Sandy Gingras, published by Down The Shore Publishing, Harvey Cedars, New Jersey (www.down-the-shore.com). Copyright © 1996 by Sandy Gingras. All rights reserved.

acknowledgments

First and foremost, I would like to say a great big thank you to my son, Cole, for his love, prayers, and extreme patience throughout the writing process for this book. He has wisdom beyond his years.

My mom, Virginia F. Nehring, who stood by my side while I adjusted to being a new mom and author both for the second time. Her undying support and unconditional love made those rough days doable.

Thanks to my sister Karen (aka Muska Puska), for her listening ears and loving heart.

I also wish to thank Roseann Caliento, my soul-friend and staunch supporter; Connie Peterson, whose friendship and thoughtfulness I treasure; and Lisa Knox, for sharing her gifts, understanding, and knowledge.

Thanks to my literary agent, who taught me so much about the world of publishing through his quiet, patient manner. I thank him for being the yin to my yang. My publicist of Teak Media Communications, who is a true blessing in my life. Her support, expertise, and friendship are always uplifting. Thanks to Andrea D'Iorio, for her awesome job of getting me to be where I need to be, so I can say what needs to be said!

Dr. Robert Robinson who shared with me strategies to make my life a positive experience. Michael Elkin, who has helped me understand how my parts make up my wholeness and who understands how humor can defuse even the most difficult situation. Dr. Ali Domar for being a powerful force for couples experiencing infertility and her support of my endeavors. Dr. Donald Moine for sharing his knowledge. Dan Sullivan of the Strategic Coach Program, who has helped me indirectly through Mark's sharing from his programs.

I thank Molly Mullen Ward, my witty, wonderful editor and champion of this book and the issue of infertility. She made this book a reality. Thanks also to Paula Decker for making the editing process smooth and complete and to Lauren Lawson for her public relations expertise.

Lastly, thanks to my daughter, Gracie, and my husband, Mark. It was an extraordinary experience growing up together while writing this book.

And thank you to all the unmentioned angels that helped in one form or another along the way. I send my thanks to you and to God for his support.

I'm grateful for all of your presences in my life. My love to you all!

American Infertility Association
666 Fifth Avenue, Suite 278
New York, NY 10103
info@americaninfertility.org
(888) 917-3777
(718) 621-5083
www.americaninfertility.org

American Society for Reproductive Medicine
(Formerly the American Fertility Society)
1209 Montgomery Highway
Birmingham, AL 35216-2809
(205) 978-5000
(205) 978-5005
www.asrm.org

RESOLVE: The National Infertility Association
1310 Broadway, Somerville, MA 02144
Business Office: 617-623-1156
Toll-Free HelpLine: 888-623-0744
info@resolve.org
www.resolve.org

Suggested Reading

Conquering Infertility: Dr. Alice Domar's Mind/Body Guide to Enhancing Fertility and Coping With Infertility, Alice D. Domar, Ph.D. and Alice Lesch Kelly

The Couple's Guide to Fertility, Gary S. Berger, M.D., Marc Goldstein, M.D., and Mark Fuerst

Experiencing Infertility: An Essential Resource, Debby Peoples and Harriette Rovner Ferguson

Girlfriend to Girlfriend: A Fertility Companion, Kristen Magnacca

The Wellness Book: The Comprehensive Guide to Maintaining Health and Treating Stress-Related Illness, Herbert Benson, M.D. and Eileen M. Stuart, R.N.C., M.S.

Web Support

www.fertility.com
www.seronofertility.com
www.fertilityneighborhood.com
https://fertility.webmd.com

D

deal-making, 167, 169–170

Domar, Ali, 7–8, 32, 48, 161

Dreams List, 3–10; putting
into practice, 9–10

Ducking and Dodging, 82–87,
91

E

Einstein, Albert, 108

"Elevator Speech," 79–81,
134, 145

Encarta World English Dictionary, 114

F

Fertility Game Plan, 11–19,
74; putting into practice,
17–19; reasons to have,
14; samples of, 15–17

Fertility Log, 51–53

filling jar, 148–151, 170

Firewalk, 181, 182

G

Gingras, Sandy, 182

*Girlfriend to Girlfriend: A Fer-
tility Companion* (Mag-
nacca), 66

gratitude. *See also* Gratitude
List: celebrating victories
and, 179–180; gratitude
principle and, 177

Gratitude List, 39–43, 178;
abundance and, 46; as
complement to journaling,
41, 43, 178; putting into
practice, 43

Gray, John, 87, 168

groups of couples that enter
parenthood, xi–xii. *See also*
"one enchanted evening"
pregnancy group

H

Hawn, Goldie, 165

Hill, Napoleon, 10

Holmes, Oliver Wendell, 39

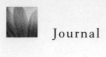

Journal

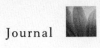

Journal

Journal

Journal

Journal

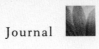

Journal